Tongue Tie

from confusion to clarity

a guide to the diagnosis

and treatment of

Ankyloglossia

(Tongue Tie)

CARMEN FERNANDO LCST MSPAA
Speech Pathologist

FOREWORD BY DR MARTIN GLASSON FRCS FRACS
Head, Douglas Cohen Department of Paediatric Surgery
New Children's Hospital, Westmead NSW Australia

TANDEM PUBLICATIONS
Sydney, Australia

Note to Readers:
For consistency, the term 'patient' has been used throughout this
book in preference to 'client' since most of the subjects had hospital
treatment. The anonymity of patients has been preserved by not using
their real names.

First published in 1998 by
Tandem Publications
28 Macnamara Avenue
CONCORD NSW 2137
Australia

Telephone: +61 2 9746 2745

**National Library of Australia
Cataloguing-in-Publication data:**

Fernando, Carmen.
Tongue tie—from confusion to clarity: a guide to
the diagnosis and treatment of ankyloglossia.

Bibliography.
Includes index.
ISBN 0 646 35254 7.

1. Ankyloglossia. 2. Ankyloglossia - Case studies.
3. Lingual frenum - Surgery.

616.8550436

Photographs used for Plates 1-24 by courtesy of
New Children's Hospital, Westmead, New South Wales

Printed in Australia by Australian Print Group, Maryborough, Victoria

Design and typesetting by Sue Rawkins Design

Foreword

With tongue tie (ankyloglossia), the fraenum linguae is short, tight and often fan-shaped and as a consequence the tongue is bound down to the floor of the mouth. Traditional teaching expressed both in medical texts and in guidebooks for young parents has been that tongue tie is of little relevance, will have no adverse sequelae, and can be ignored.

Over the past two decades the truth has emerged: tongue tie, by interfering with tongue mobility, can exert a harmful effect upon many aspects of life. Speech might develop abnormally because the tip of the tongue needs to be placed upon the roof of the mouth to produce some sounds. Dental hygiene is restricted because of limited access of the tongue to the back of the mouth. Functions dependent upon protrusion of the tongue (including, for a child, the licking of an ice cream) are inhibited. Along with this has come the realisation that the quality of life of patients with tongue tie can be improved by an operation which is simple, brief and virtually devoid of complications.

Carmen Fernando in her work as a speech pathologist has developed a particular interest and expertise in tongue tie and its impact on speech. Her contributions have been of great importance in the process of overturning the previous incorrect beliefs concerning the significance of tongue tie. In this definitive monograph she draws upon her wealth of experience to describe every aspect of tongue tie in painstaking detail. It will interest health professionals who work with children and should be mandatory reading for all speech pathologists, whether in training or in practice.

MARTIN GLASSON

New Children's Hospital
Westmead NSW 2145
Australia

This book is dedicated to
the 256 patients with tongue tie
who contributed to the study
which led to the findings
detailed herein.

Contents

Preface   vii
1. Introduction   **1**

2. Historical background   **4**
  Early references   4
  Contemporary references   4
  Changing attitudes   5
  Criteria for surgery   6

3. The hidden agenda of tongue tie   **7**
  Feeding difficulty   8
  Oral hygiene, dental health and dentition   9
  Uncontrolled salivation   10
  The tongue-thrust swallow   11
  Impaired tongue mobility   12
  Speech impairment   12
  Lowered self esteem   13

4. Assessment criteria   **17**
  Devising assessment measures   17
  Objectives of assessment   18
  The method devised   19
  Case history   19
  Importance of visual assessment   20
  The seven criteria   20

5. Surgery for tongue tie   **28**
  Can surgery help?   28
  When surgery is recommended   28
  Conflicting priorities   29
  The operation then and now   30
  The surgical procedure   30
  Recovery after surgery   31
  Discomfort after surgery   32
  Aiming for optimal surgery   32
  Post-operative findings   33

6. Speech therapy after surgery   **34**
   The critical age   35
   Late operation   35
   After surgery   36
   Post-operative follow-up   36
   Oral hygiene   37
   Feeding   37
   Lingual movements   38
   Oral kinaesthesia   38
   Speech   38
   Therapeutic prognosis   39
   When intensive therapy is required   40

7. Case histories   **41**
   Introduction   41
   Case history 1: Optimal management   42
     of tongue tie
   Case history 2: A mild tie that proved to   43
     be significant
   Case history 3: The long and the short of it!   46
   Case history 4: Conflicting priorities   48
   Case history 5: Delayed intervention delivers   50
     limited success
   Case history 6: Practice makes perfect   52
   Case history 7: A quantum leap may occur ...   54
   Case history 8: Expect the unexpected   56
   Case history 9: When you can't see the wood   58
     for the trees
   Case history 10: Keeping a stiff upper lip   60

Appendix A Summary of the study   62
Appendix B Assessing ankyloglossia   64
Appendix C Surgical procedures   72
Appendix D Exercises for improving lingual   74
   proficiency
References   83
Glossary   85
Index   87

ILLUSTRATIONS
Plates *(between pages 40 and 41)*
Figure D1 Section of oral cavity   74

Preface

Ankyloglossia, often referred to as 'tongue tie', could be called the Cinderella of speech therapy—mistreated, misunderstood and ignored. It usually occurs in close conjunction with a question mark, and its incidence in the population is as yet unknown.

This book has been written in the hope that it will help show how ankyloglossia can be recognised, assessed, understood and managed with confidence.

In 1981, while working as a speech pathologist at the Royal Alexandra Hospital for Children in Sydney, I was asked to look into the question of why so many children were being referred to the Speech Pathology department for opinions as to the need for tongue tie surgery. Although the condition was generally considered to be insignificant, parents were consistently experiencing difficulties and were seeking help. We were aware that some of these children had long standing speech problems. Others had been referred from overseas and were returning to situations where speech pathology was not available.

When a search of the literature produced only a small number of articles on the subject, it was decided to embark on a study of all the children being referred to the hospital with the diagnosis of tongue tie, and thereby to acquire some current data. We planned to accumulate information indiscriminately— in the hope of eventually sifting out significant features.

In May 1983 a paper was presented to the Australian College of Paediatrics' Annual Conference in Brisbane with the conclusion that surgery was often an appropriate form of intervention for tongue tie. The proposition provoked considerable controversy. This was partly because the need for another surgical procedure, tonsillectomy, was currently under scrutiny, and partly because the prevailing thought on tongue tie was that it had to be extremely severe to warrant surgical release.

By October 1997, at the Royal Alexandra Hospital for Children and in my private practice, I had collected data on 256 patients with tongue tie and my earlier conclusion regarding the validity of the surgical option in cases of tongue tie was further substantiated (a summary of the study is given in Appendix A).

At this time I had also developed a simple assessment procedure, the Tongue tie Assessment Protocol or TAP, to determine whether surgery was warranted. This protocol was used to assess all patients referred with a diagnosis of possible tongue tie. Two hundred of these patients for whom complete records were available have been included in the study.

The 13 patients who had surgery and were included in the original presentation in May 1983 formed the nucleus of the larger group of 200 now being discussed. Of this group of 200 patients with tongue tie, surgery was recommended for 196 patients. Only 175 patients—approximately 87% of the group—finally had surgery. All the patients who were operated on were followed up and further assessments made with TAP after surgery, and after speech therapy, when the latter was indicated. Invariably, a substantial measurable improvement was seen after intervention.

Those patients who decided against surgery often did not persevere with therapy, and those who had therapy alone did not achieve the desired results.

The purpose of this book is to enumerate the many factors involved with tongue tie, to describe presenting symptoms (assisted by the inclusion of 24 colour plates), to show that surgery is appropriate in many cases and that the optimal management of tongue tie requires the services of both surgeon and speech pathologist in very specific ways.

The use of the assessment protocol TAP, based on seven criteria, is fully explained to enable speech pathologists to use this tool in a combined assessment and management plan, which has the potential for highly successful outcomes. This observation is firmly based on the improvement seen in speech and lifestyle for the majority of patients in the study.

I wish to express my sincere appreciation of the support and encouragement received from Dr Martin Glasson, without whose help the study would not have commenced. Dr Glasson's generous advice, assistance and expertise in this small but significant clinical area have made a considerable impact on the project. I also acknowledge the contributions from Dr Edward Beckenham and Dr Hugh Martin who made available a description of their procedures for tongue-tie surgery for inclusion in the book. The success of the surgical results has contributed in great measure to our understanding of this topic.

I am grateful to Wendy Sinclair for her meticulous editing of the manuscript, to Pixie Maloney for taking the photographs for Plates 1 to 24, to Robyn Murrell for initiating the study, to Anne Lyon for keeping records, to Alison McKeown for her suggestions, to Shamin Fernando for taking the photographs for Plates 25-31 and for the illustration, to Dayanthi and Mark Bonarius, Michelle Fernando and Greg Hassall for their assistance with the many tasks involved with writing and publishing this book.

Finally, and most importantly, I wish to thank my husband Lalin, for his encouragement and practical help, his computer literacy, and his patience.

1   Introduction

Tongue tie is one of the oldest known anatomical defects affecting speech. A Biblical reference to tongue tie reads: '… and the bond which tied his tongue was loosed, and he talked plainly.' Mark 7:35.

While this topic has never been comprehensively investigated, tongue tie has occasionally been written-up in medical journals as an interesting phenomenon. It is well known, for instance, that tongue tie frequently occurs in association with other congenital conditions such as cleft palate, sublingual cysts and anomalies of bony structure. While these syndromes themselves have been well researched, the implications for patients with tongue tie have been largely ignored.

Although tongue tie has tended to be regarded as a minor problem, Greene[1] estimates that 0.2 to 0.3 per 1000 of the population has tongue tie. Of course, much depends on how these figures are derived—at what age the patient is diagnosed, and what criteria are used for making the diagnosis.

Speech pathologists and patients are therefore justified in being confused as to how this condition should be viewed. Certainly, it does exist. Oldfield writing in the *Lancet* in 1955 stated unequivocally: 'These babies can be seen nearly every week in the out-patient department of any big hospital. The degree of disability is variable and debatable, but not the existence of the deformity.'[2]

Ketty and Sciullo[3] state that early studies by DePorte and Parkhurst[4] and McEnery and Gaines[5] report the incidence of ankyloglossia to be 0.4 per 1000, and 4 per 1000 of the population, respective-

ly, but later studies by Schaumann[6] and Witkop[7] give the incidence as 22 and 68.3 per 1000, respectively.

The variations are acknowledged and explained thus: 'Because there is no standardised definition of a tongue tie condition, meaningful prevalence studies are not available.'[8] Incidences ranging from 99 out of 273,600 births[4] to 0.2 or 0.3 per 1000 of the population[1] have been suggested.

These figures, however, are misleading and add to the confusion prevailing around the topic of tongue tie. Williams and Waldron have described the various aspects which authors have focussed upon when defining tongue tie:

> Some authors have defined tongue tie as a lingual frenulum that is short, thick, or fibrosed; others have defined it as a condition in which the tongue is actually fused to the floor of the mouth. Still other definitions have emphasised specific disorders (dental, skeletal, and speech) related to the tongue tie rather than defining the degree of lingual restriction … Again, lack of a common definition and objective measurements has prevented the identification of any true relationship between tongue tie and speech disorders.[8]

A retrospective study was performed by Dr James Wright of Newcastle, Australia, and reported in 1995. He distinguishes between 'simple tongue-tie' and 'true ankyloglossia'; patients with the latter condition being excluded from the study. Here again, the problem of definition arises—diagnosis being based on a reliance on physical appearance only, rather than on both appearance and function. He concluded that 'speech difficulties related to tongue-tie are over-rated and mechanical problems are under-estimated."[9]

As a result of information gathered in the course of my study, I have formulated my own definition of the condition based on both visual and functional aspects of the frenum:

Tongue tie is a congenital condition, recognised by an unusually thickened, tightened or shortened frenum, which limits movement of the tongue in activities connected with feeding and which has an adverse impact on both dental health and speech.

However it may have been defined, over the past 50 years it has been the custom for various health professionals to state that tongue tie very rarely requires surgical intervention. Many and varied reasons have been proffered for this attitude. For instance, degrees of lingual limitation which permit protrusion of the tongue tip to the vermilion, or downward protrusion towards the chin, or which allow so-called 'active movement', are all deemed insignificant and unlikely to affect speech production. Another view is that a tie is worthy of surgical intervention only if it prevents feeding, or if speech is grossly affected—with defective articulation of several single sounds. The common theme is to avoid recommending surgery.

Fletcher and Meldrum, writing in the *Journal of Speech and Hearing* in 1968, made this striking observation:

> … the incidence of this anatomical restriction and it's specific physiological effect are conjectural in spite of written interest and speculation in this topic which spans several hundred years (Dessantz, 1760, von Rosenstein, 1776, Moss, 1794, Cullum, 1959, Tuerk and Lubit, 1959, Spitzer, 1960).[10]

It is impossible to predict accurately how much disability will result from any particular untreated tongue tie. The vast range of movements possible to healthy lingual musculature, gives the individ-

ual the capability for much variation in the field of communication. Oral musculature, intonation, body language and gesture can be used to complement speech, and can result in real physiological problems being camouflaged, so that patients do not receive the treatment that would benefit them. Speech pathologists are familiar with the devices of concealment that people who stutter, for instance, employ to avoid being identified as having a speech problem. Patients with tongue tie also attempt to mask their problems, and often fail to be diagnosed.

Fletcher and Meldrum wrote:

> … for many years "folk thinking" concerning errors of speech placed heavy emphasis upon freedom of lingual movement. The speech specialist and various medical specialists recognised the futility of routinely "clipping the tongue" and waged a successful battle against lingual surgery for speech disorders. The question which was not answered in this foray was, "What is the relationship which exists between lingual mobility and speech proficiency?"[10]

They go on to show that one condition affects the other.

Every patient with suspected tongue tie must be looked at individually. Patients respond to limitation in their own way—tolerating, mastering or compensating in ways that suit the individual's personality. It is vital, therefore, that speech pathologists learn to recognise and assess the appearance and movements of tongues in the light of theoretical knowledge about tongue tie.

As with other speech pathologies, early diagnosis and well planned management are extremely important. As a result of the clinical work I have done with patients who have tongue tie and patients with other speech defects, I do not see any validity in 'wait and see' policies. If the patient is experiencing disability because of a tongue tie—as shown by assessment—and is strong enough to handle surgery and capable of benefiting from the advantages it offers (i.e. the patient has no other severe physical or developmental disabilities), I recommend that surgery be carried out.

Currently, because of earlier prejudice against diagnosing tongue tie, the condition is often overlooked. Consequently, prolonged therapy may be embarked upon to correct what is, after all, an anatomical defect. The degree of the defect, as well as the history and circumstances of the patient, determine the impact of the condition on the individual, as with any other speech problem.

The following comment, made after comparing diadochokinetic movements and sublingual dimensions in 40 children in the 11 to 12-year-old age group, merits consideration by speech pathologists:

> Perhaps in discarding an unwarranted over-generalisation concerning "tongue tie" and speech articulation [that tongue tie never causes speech problems], speech clinicians have overlooked a potentially fruitful clinical consideration which may, in fact, help to clarify certain types of disorders of speech and other biological functions of the mouth.[10]

Even though the expression 'tongue-tied' has passed into our language as signifying halting, arrhythmic or ineffective speech, the physical, social and emotional implications of this condition have been largely ignored.

However, until tongue tie is accepted as a significant pathological condition with far reaching negative consequences for those who have it and for their families, it is unlikely that researchers will address the question of its prevalence, or its effects on the population.

The benefits experienced by the patients in my study who had surgery have demonstrated the need to rethink old attitudes in the light of methodical assessment procedures. The study results have not justified the practice of denying surgery to patients with tongue tie on the basis of old-established theories and hopeful prognostications.

The propensity to put off surgical intervention in the hope that the patient will adjust to the disability is equally disastrous, because the best effects are achieved by surgery before poor speech habits can be formed.

It is clear that where effective treatment exists for any disability it behoves us to administer it, rather than to wait in the hope that it will not be needed. It may be argued that this is especially so when the treatment in question is a minor procedure, offering a quick recovery period and little risk.

2 Historical Background

References dating back to biblical times point to tongue tie as an anatomical defect occurring persistently across social and ethnic boundaries and recognise its medical and social significance. In early times it was not considered to be a controversial issue and was dealt with promptly by practical, though not always sophisticated, measures.

EARLY REFERENCES

In the 1600s, midwives kept a fingernail sharp in case it might be necessary to tear the frenum of a newborn infant. A publication in 1697 contained the following advice under the heading 'Of loosening the string of the tongue, and of the ranula under the tongue':

> It happens often in infants, that the tongue is bound so straight by the string, that it cannot well or freely move and sometimes in the place where the bridle of the tongue is, a soft and white swelling appears, which they call the Ranula.
>
> The binding of the tongue is most conveniently removed by surgery; for though midwives often break the string as soon as the child is born, or cut it with a groat, yet they often err in the operation, and do it many times when there is no occasion, therefore it is much safer to use a skilful surgeon; afterwards apply the following linament.[11]

Concern regarding the lack of hygiene and safety in such methods led to the invention of the 'grooved director' in the seventeenth century by Petit, a French surgeon. This instrument protects the blood vessels at the base of the tongue from accidental injury when the frenum is clipped and was included in standard surgical equipment.

In 1729, *The Nurses' Guide, or the Right Method of Bringing Up Young Children* stated unequivocally that a short membrane under the tongue hinders a child from sucking. In a passage 'concerning such defects as children often bring with them out of their mothers' womb into the world which ought to be rectified with all speed,' it states that: 'Very often the membrane under the tongue is so short and strait [sic] that it hinders the child from sucking and puts him in a condition of never being able to speak distinctly all his life, but these inconveniences are easily removed by a slight incision.'[12]

CONTEMPORARY REFERENCES

Until the early twentieth century, even professionals tended to attribute all speech problems including stuttering, lisping and delayed development of speech, to tongue tie. In the folk tales of many countries tongue tie is mentioned. Indeed, midwives in many rural communities are still accustomed to checking babies at birth and, when considered necessary, to separate the frenum themselves. Middle European parents are particularly critical of untreated tongue tie as it is a routine procedure in their home communities for these to be freed at birth.

There are contemporary literary references to tongue tie as a medical condition. In Maxine Hong Kingston's autobiographical novel *The Woman*

Warrior—Memoirs of a Girlhood among Ghosts the author mentions how her mother, a woman doctor in China, cut the frenum of her tongue. Her mother explains: 'I cut it so that you would not be tongue-tied. Your tongue would be able to move in any language.'[13]

Ankyloglossia is often listed as a congenital disorder of the tongue. Isaac van der Waal defines it as '... a congenital developmental condition in which the tongue is abnormally fixed to the floor of the mouth or the lingual aspect of the gingival mucosa (or both) because of a short and malpositioned frenulum linguae.'[14]

There were several instances of family histories of tongue tie among the patients in my study, and it often happened that a sibling, parent, grandparent or other relative was reported as having similar symptoms. Unlike the younger patients, these older family members had been readily diagnosed as having a problem, although they might not have received any treatment. Once methodical prevalence studies have established the incidence of tongue tie in the population it will be possible to evaluate the significance of the genetic factor in tongue tie.

In 1959 an English surgeon, Dennis Browne, described a case of familial tongue tie in the *British Medical Journal*: 'One of my cases had the family history that the father had been wasting away as a small baby till an aged midwife produced a scissors from her pocket and cut the frenulum there and then, with the result that he put on a pound in the next few days.'[15]

However, in recent literature it is only rarely that feeding difficulties, and in particular breast-feeding difficulties, are attributed to tongue tie.

CHANGING ATTITUDES

This change of attitude has a historical basis. In the period 1830 to 1841 a great wave of surgery swept over France, Germany and England.

Deiffenbach in Germany, Yearsley and Braid in England and Velpeau in France saw surgery as the ultimate cure for many types of ailments. In 1841, 200 stutterers were treated with surgery, and strange operations—including the removal of the uvula for a cough—were being performed with no beneficial effects for the patient.

When the swing of the pendulum occurred, a wave of revulsion swept over Europe and the number of operations performed declined markedly. Surgery for tongue tie has been in limbo ever since.

It was probably no coincidence that when bottle feeding came into vogue in the 1930s,[16] attitudes unfavourable to surgical treatment of tongue tie also became the custom. While a breastfed infant needs to coordinate his tongue—by placing and moving it as part of an effectively functioning oral sucking machine—a bottle–fed baby might feed acceptably with incorrect movements, since compression of the rubber nipple by any means would deliver the milk.

The standpoint of most speech pathologists during the 1950s was that it was not a condition that required surgery unless the severity of the tie was such that it interfered with feeding and caused malnourishment. Such severe ties were, however, difficult to identify, as many mothers learn to feed their children despite physical problems by a combination of determination, skill and luck.

Mothers who insisted that their children had tongue ties were looked upon as fussy, neurotic or over-protective, and surgery for tongue tie became increasingly unfashionable. Surgeons who were willing to perform the operation needed unquestionable justification before they would agree to intervene.

In 1968 Jean R Block, writing about indications for surgery, specified these instances where surgery was not recommended:

(1) if there is a short frenulum, but tongue tip sounds are not affected, then frenulotomy would not be supported,
(2) if tongue tip sounds are produced incorrectly, but the individual can be stimulated to produce these sounds, frenulotomy would not be indicated on the basis of speech production.[17]

In 1972, Muriel Morley wrote:

This condition is frequently blamed for defective articulation. It is however possible for speech to be normal to the casual ear when there is a severe degree of tongue tie.[18]

She implies, somewhat ambiguously, that the speech one hears is not the effortless process it may seem to be to the casual listener.

CRITERIA FOR SURGERY
As a result of these circumstances, for at least 100 years surgical intervention in cases of tongue tie has been unpopular. Definitions of the condition vary from one authority to the next, and there is no consensus of opinion as to the criteria for recommending surgery, or the optimal age for performing it.

In 1963, Antony Wallace gave this opinion on surgical intervention:

No frenulum should be divided before the age of four years, and thereafter only if the mechanism of tongue protrusion is too feeble to stretch or rupture it (Smithells 1959). Even after division, defective articulation will probably persist. A healthy intelligent child, more than four years of age and with a persistent tongue tie, is very uncommon.[19]

However, by the age of four the child with tongue tie would have built up very strong habits of oromuscular function, based on the limited tongue movements available to him or her. If speech were considered the major criterion for a recommendation of surgery, a tongue tie could not be diagnosed for several years, by which time patterns of oromuscular functioning would be well established, and correspondingly hard to correct. The detrimental effects of delayed intervention on oromuscular function in children with tongue tie has attracted the attention of various professionals. Nurses, dentists and paediatricians have observed negative effects on feeding, dental health and speech—all powerful arguments in favour of early intervention.

3   The Hidden Agenda of Tongue Tie

Information gathered for the study from scrutiny of the available literature offered many different points of view—but few answers. The most obvious questions are still being asked, such as:

- Does the condition exist?
- If so, is ankyloglossia the same as tongue tie?
- Is ankyloglossia simply a more severe form of tongue tie?
- Should a surgical remedy be prescribed?
- If so, when?
- Are feeding difficulties and speech impairment the only factors that should determine the need for surgery?

As my study progressed, it became apparent that there are many more facets to this condition than the much-canvassed aspects already detailed. There are more poignant limitations than the often-quoted inability to play a wind instrument which was mentioned by Antony Wallace in his letter to the Lancet in 1963.[19] In fact, there is a 'hidden agenda' to tongue tie which operates in every case, to a greater or lesser degree, and unless all aspects of this condition are considered, we will not have a full understanding of the extent to which tongue tie can affect the functioning of patients. If we have only a limited understanding of the condition, we are not in a position to offer solutions.

During the study many parents, dentists and relatives offered information and anecdotes about tongue tie. This anecdotal data was reinforced by:

- similarities between the presenting symptoms of patients;
- clinical observations of patients currently having therapy; and
- reported and observed symptoms of adult relatives with tongue tie.

The difficulties experienced embraced pronunciation, quality of speech under stress, lack of control of rapid speech, unpleasant cosmetic appearance of the tongue, apparent hypersalivation (which was actually the result of ineffective swallowing) and immediate deterioration of speech if the patient indulged in even the smallest amount of alcohol.

Some adults in the study reported negative comments from listeners including: 'Why can't you speak when you are angry?'; 'You are lazy'; 'Have you got a split tongue?'; 'You sound like a cockatoo'; and 'He has a forked tongue.'

One mother described her newborn as having a 'serpent's tongue'. Another described her baby when breastfeeding as a 'barracuda biting at the breast'.

Adult relatives spoke of the way they had adapted to the difficulties of pronouncing certain speech sounds, and described such tricks as clicking or sucking on the palate to substitute for a T or D sound. These techniques may have provided a substitute, but they also made the adult's speech both unclear and conspicuous.

Effects on feeding and speech are predictable, but the patients seen showed a much broader spectrum of disability—some typical case histories have been included in Chapter 7.

FEEDING DIFFICULTY

An important function of the tongue is, of course, its use in feeding, and, when the tongue performs well in vegetative functions, it provides the basis for good oromuscular function in speech. This has been a fundamental tenet of speech pathology from its inception. Today, however, many professionals do not acknowledge the severe detrimental effects of tongue tie on feeding. While conceding that tongue tie caused some other problems, Dr Ian Kern of Sydney, Australia, writing in the Medical Journal of Australia, stated that: 'In infancy, tongue tie never causes feeding problems ...'[20]

Professor J K Barclay of Dunedin, New Zealand, writing in Patient Management, expressed a similar opinion: '... tongue-tie is seldom detected during infancy as there is no interference with suckling and eating.'[21]

Dr James Wright of Newcastle, Australia, feels that 'There may be rare instances in infancy where problems with feeding and suction can be helped by frenulotomy but evidence for this is anecdotal.'[9]

However, there are several contrary opinions and some of these are detailed below.

Breastfeeding

The following comment came from Margaret McDonald, a midwife who has studied breastfeeding difficulties in infants with physical abnormalities of the mouth:

> Whilst most of the current literature states that tongue tie does not affect feeding, the experience of mothers nursing infants with a tongue tie has been one of inability to achieve correct attachment, poor milk exchange and nipple trauma.[22]

Virginia Thorley, a lactation consultant, describes two instances of mothers receiving severe abrasions of the nipple through faulty suck, one of which involved a baby with tongue tie.[23] She has developed a technique for correcting a faulty suck.

Lactation consultants have found that some babies with tongue tie will try a number of compensatory movements of the oral musculature to achieve suckling, and this incorrect pattern of movement becomes a habit. However, as explained by Gregory Notestine, it remains an incorrect habit, since the tongue cannot extend to cover the gumline in sucking and the breastfeeding mother may suffer nipple damage, pain or mastitis during ineffective suckling attempts.[24]

These consultants maintain that even when the frenum is separated, suck training is needed unless the operation has been done within hours of birth. It is therefore salutary to ponder on what might be the consequences of long-delayed operations on speech patterns.

The undulating, wavelike movements of infantile sucking cannot be made in the presence of tongue tie. Instead of compressing the milk reservoirs, the anterior part of the tongue rubs against the nipple and presses it against the hard palate. The nipple is then in a position to be damaged by repeated 'chomping' between the gums, for the tongue tie prevents the front of the tongue from masking the lower gum ridge and protecting the nipple area.

Information derived from my study showed that 20 per cent of mothers had difficulty breastfeeding. If the mother's breast was small, highly elastic and had milk reservoirs close to the nipple, the baby might tap these with little apparent difficulty. However, nipple problems that occurred were often serious enough to stop breastfeeding. Scarred, cracked and bleeding nipples, infection and fever, bruising, distortion of shape after feeding, and the pain of mastitis marred the breastfeeding experience.

One mother who was a physiotherapist held her baby bolt upright when breastfeeding, and found that the baby could 'latch-on' in this position. Many mothers reported that they had to abandon breastfeeding attempts (including expressing milk) because the process was so traumatic, lengthy and unsatisfying for both baby and mother. Fidgety, fluttering, seeking movements of the baby trying to achieve 'latch-on' panicked new mothers who did not have the benefit of informed advice.

Bottle feeding and solids

Many babies also had problems with the bottle. Yet other mothers did not have difficulty feeding until the children were introduced to solids. A few mothers found that posture feeding helped them.

A small number of mothers found that their babies choked and gagged so much on supplements and solids, that they could only be breast-fed—therefore for the purpose of nourishment these babies were still being breastfed at 2 years and 9 months!

As observed in the case of older patients with eating problems, these symptoms appear to have been caused by limitation of lingual movements resulting in poor oral kinaesthesia.

The baby with tongue tie is only capable of a small range of tongue movements. This infant cannot elevate the tongue tip to the hard palate when the lower jaw is dropped and often cannot coordinate the retraction and elevation of the posterior part of the tongue in swallowing, because the tight lingual frenum pulls the tongue forward.

When the frenum extends right up to the tongue tip, there is, in effect, no tip; the margin of the tongue is pulled and curled under towards the buccal floor. This means that licking or lateral movements of the tongue are distorted, but may sometimes be attempted with concomitant jaw movement.

Consequences

In the long term, the most destructive aspect of this situation is that the tongue is incapable of exploring the oral cavity, and because of this loss of experimentation, the baby cannot cope with change in the oral area. New movements, or unfamiliar textures—substances, spoons, teats, or unusual amounts of milk flowing into the mouth—will be perceived as unwelcome. Until the baby has familiarised itself with coordination of the new movements needed to deal with breast, bottle or spoon-feeding, there will be difficulty.

Mothers frequently mentioned that children with tongue tie had poor chewing and swallowing habits; food was often gulped down with drinks of water, or not accepted unless it was of a soft or easily chewable texture. Food debris was often noted around the mouth after a meal, and in some cases remained in the cheek pouches and between the teeth. One mother of a 10-month-old boy had to check her son's mouth routinely after a meal and at bed time for leftovers, which she frequently found.

Many children with tongue tie had a history of frequent upper respiratory tract infection and regurgitation and several were treated for gastro-oesophageal reflux. It is arguable that these conditions could have been exacerbated by food debris remaining in the mouth after feeds and subsequently being aspirated.

ORAL HYGIENE, DENTAL HEALTH AND DENTITION

Another serious consequence of tongue tie is its contribution to poor oral and dental hygiene. This has been convincingly proved by dental experts but, strangely, this factor does not appear to have carried much weight with other professionals.

Professor Barclay comments: '… the tongue is unable to clear food from the buccal sulci, and if good oral hygiene is not practised, carious lesions may develop on the buccal aspect of the teeth.'[21]

Ketty has reported 'periodontal pockets and gingival recession in the region of the mandibular incisors'[25] in six out of 24 cases of ankyloglossia.

Some controversy has also arisen about the extent to which abnormal tongue movements can affect the shape or position of bony structures in the mouth, and as to whether the tongue-thrusting during swallowing that is often seen in these patients is a cause or an effect of dental malocclusion, lisping and lateralisation of sibilants.

When considering patients with cleft palate and cerebral palsy, the structure and functioning of the mouth is accepted as being of major importance in remediation. Yet the limitation of lingual movement consequent upon tongue tie is apparently not seen as a problem that should be remediable by surgery, unless in cases of extreme severity.

Dental problems are identified by Whitman and Rankow:

> ... perverted use of the tongue is a very prevalent factor in certain types of malocclusion ... fibres of the genioglossus muscle are too short or they are attached in such a way that the tongue is held too low in the mouth, giving the appearance of macroglossia ... In many instances the upper arch is under-developed and the lower arch is over-developed because of the abnormally low position of the tongue. If the tongue is held a little higher in the mouth, a lateral tongue thrust may be present thus causing an open bite ... on one or both sides. The characteristic rest position is one in which the tongue spreads out laterally, and ... the pressure of the tongue is upward against the maxillary buccal teeth and downwards against the mandibular buccal teeth. This prevents these teeth from erupting to their full occlusal height ... the appearance is that of a deep overbite. If the tongue is held somewhat higher and protruded ... there is an anterior open bite.[26]

Many children in my study who were over the age of 7 years had dental caries. Under this age tooth brushing is usually supervised, and fluoride in the drinking water provides some protection.

Several mothers found that they had to check their children's mouths after meals to make sure that all food had been swallowed. In one large general hospital in Sydney, dental surgeons insist on carrying out tongue tie surgery because they are so concerned about the detrimental effects of the tie on the dental health of the patient.

The difficulty patients experience in manipulating the bolus of food during mastication and swallowing results in food particles getting lodged in hard-to-reach parts of the mouth. Consideration of the significant limitation of elevation, retraction, protrusion, circular and lateral tongue movements in patients with tongue tie will show that retrieval of shreds of food, if attempted, will be inefficient.

One 5-year-old child seen had had both upper and lower incisors filled under general anaesthetic. However the fillings deteriorated quickly and were repeated, again under a general anaesthetic.

Due to poor oral kinaesthetic sense, it is likely that the patient is less aware of food debris in the mouth and will not locate it easily. Food stuck to the palate will be inaccessible. Decaying of stale food will cause the development of plaque and, subsequently, caries and gingivitis. Retrieval of food lost between the lips and teeth can risk injury to the frenum and excessive effort can repeatedly rupture it. However, that effort is seldom made spontaneously, and consequently oral hygiene suffers.

UNCONTROLLED SALIVATION

Poor control of saliva, causing dribbling and 'splashing' during speech is another very common consequence of tongue tie. Inefficient disposal of saliva secreted during speech and feeding can result in a very messy, wet, facial appearance. While not affecting dental health, it certainly has social repercussions and also gives rise to rashes around the mouth in both young and older children.

One patient was penalised by being excluded from school because of complaints from parents of other children, who harboured unfounded fears that the child had an infectious condition. This experience was very distressing for the patient.

The coordination of speaking and controlling salivation is a task that increases in difficulty as the sentence structure becomes more complex. Under conditions where emotion, competing noise or haste apply, the task of swallowing while maintaining precise articulatory contacts often becomes impossible.

Some children solve this dilemma by using short utterances; others talk softly and slowly. Many use a very small oral aperture and allow the saliva to pool in the mouth where it interferes with clarity and frequently spills out.

Demands that the child swallow frequently result in a slow, noisy effort. There is often little understanding of how swallowing takes place—it is seen as something to do with a drink or food, but not with saliva.

THE TONGUE–THRUST SWALLOW

With normal development of the teeth, lips, jaw and tongue, and a good feeding pattern, the mature or adult swallow appears around the sixth month. In some individuals this does not occur— with negative consequences for speech, cosmetic appearance and, as some authorities maintain, for dental health. These children and adults retain the infantile swallowing pattern which Dworkin and Culatta describe thus:

> During infantile swallowing, anteriorly directed movements of the tongue between the gum pads are common. These movements have been related to the massiveness of the tongue within a comparatively small, edentulous cavity, and to premature oroneuromotor integration (Doty, 1968; Fletcher, 1970; Humphrey, 1970).[27]

Dworkin and Culatta refer to Fletcher, who in 1970 reviewed some of the aetiological factors of the infantile swallowing pattern which is often described as 'tongue thrusting'. These factors included genetic predisposition, oroneuromotor deficiency, abnormal skeletal dental morphology, delayed maturation or retention of the infantile suckle–swallow tongue movements, regression to a less mature phase of physiological function, and learned behaviour.

Tongue thrusting during speech and feeding was often found in the cases of ankyloglossia studied. One child, who had very poor articulation and a lateral lisp before surgery, developed frontal lisping after surgery until the tongue movements came under conscious control. This was achieved with the assistance of a short period of speech therapy.

In March 1979, Young and Sacks published the results of a study performed in Philadelphia of 24 patients referred with a diagnosis of ankyloglossia. They mention that:

> Ankyloglossia is believed by some to produce abnormal muscle pressures on the teeth and mandible and to impede the development of a mature swallowing pattern.[28]

This theory has subsequently been questioned or modified by other authorities such as Williams and Waldron who wrote:

> There is little research to support the suggestion that a restricted lingual frenulum results in anterior lingual pressures of sufficient magnitude to move teeth or bone. We have observed, however, … that a prominent lingual frenulum, although not limiting tongue movement, may dislodge an individual's lower denture whenever the tongue tip is raised.[8]

It was often found that patients over the age of six who had tongue tie and an infantile swallow also had a pronounced anterior open bite, distorted mandibular incisors and dental caries. Further research is required to ascertain the correlation between these conditions.

IMPAIRED TONGUE MOBILITY

A tongue that is limited in its movements may cause other inconveniences to its owner. In adult patients, dental plates often become dislodged, to the point where lower dentures are impractical. Some dentists will free the frenum prior to fitting the denture.

Tongue protrusion can be inadequate for satisfactory examination of the mouth and throat, and repeated trauma from friction of the frenum with the teeth during coughing can lead to physical damage such as described by Jones:

> When young children cough, they stick out their tongues. In protracted bouts of coughing, e.g. in pertussis, repeated trauma of the lingual fraenum from the lower incisors produces a curious lesion resembling an epithelioma, a firm red spherical lump 4 to 5 mm in diameter, centred on the fraenum linguae.[29]

Such a lesion was excised from the frenum of one patient in the study and similar thickenings on the frenum were observed on many adults and children with tongue tie.

Young and Sacks state:

> Tongue position is also an important factor in the development of dental and facial structures. ... patients with ankyloglossia may experience problems in (1) mastication and deglutition (2) dentition and/or (3) speech.[28]

Douglas and Kresberg describe the function of the frenum and then detail what ankyloglossia is:

> The lingual phrenum is important in various physiological functions of the tongue. Its length and place of attachment limit the movement of the tip of the tongue in speech and mastication ... Ankyloglossia is caused by a short phrenum attached far forward to the floor of the mouth or the lingual gingiva. This limits the movement of the tip of the tongue, and indirectly the movement of the entire tongue ... the lingual phrenum is not muscle tissue. It is a part of the mucosa lining the floor of the mouth and the ventral surface of the tongue.[30]

SPEECH IMPAIRMENT

The speech symptoms in people with tongue tie vary widely. Since the condition has little credibility among professionals, the speech of patients with tongue tie has not been fully researched, and the theory that only tongue-tip sounds are affected by tongue tie is based merely on deduction.

Browne describes the speech of older subjects vividly: 'In older children the effect is a curiously muffled voice that can be imitated by trying to talk with the tip of the tongue held under the lower teeth.'[15]

Observation of the patients in my study showed that speech may be affected as a result of tongue tie in one or more of the following areas:

- Clarity of pronunciation of sounds is reduced.
- Fluency in the production of speech is disrupted.
- Quality of the sound of speech is affected.

Due to the fact that co-ordination of the oral musculature in feeding and speech are the most damaging weaknesses of the patient with tongue tie, many patients had problems in more than one aspect of speech.

Pronunciation

Errors in articulation tended to be of two types: consistent inability to pronounce certain sounds; and inconsistent errors which occurred under conditions of stress, lengthy or rapid speech, or speech which was produced unusually softly or loudly. This speech was characterised by blurring of articulatory contacts, vowel changes due to altered lingual postures, distortions caused by excess of saliva in the mouth, inability to produce variations of stress in polysyllabic words, and less frequently, prolongations of final continuant consonants. Most patients also tended to maintain a small oral opening when speaking—thus muffling their speech further.

It was found that traditional symptom-oriented therapy had to be augmented by work done on the particular weaknesses of patients with tongue tie, however successful the surgery had been, if progress was to be achieved with the older patient. This is another argument in favour of early diagnosis and remediation.

Fluency

Disruption of fluency was often found with the speech of many patients being arrhythmic, jerky, abrupt, drawling or slow. In a small number of cases where there was a family history of stuttering, the patient with tongue tie also stuttered. This suggested to me that the frustration of limited lingual mobility and poor communication might have triggered or precipitated an incipient stutter.

Quality

Dysphonia was frequently found as a result of effortful or forced voicing but this quickly improved after surgery if the habit had not become too firmly entrenched. The problem of forced voicing seems to arise as a result of tension and efforts to compensate for unclear articulation.

In some instances, the child was attempting to compete with assertive siblings who were unhandicapped by speech problems. Being unable to discriminate kinaesthetically between precise articulatory contacts and forced sounds, and often being unable to achieve the contacts in connected speech, the child would become accustomed to forcing his voice. This symptom abated without specific therapy, following surgery.

Involuntary pitch changes and intermittent hypernasality under stress were often found, and when these were present in older children, were of

course more difficult to eradicate. In three of the patients seen, the degree of distortion of speech as a result was quite severe.

One child I saw at the age of five had completed 2 years of speech therapy but was still frequently unintelligible in connected speech. The tongue tie looked only moderately severe cosmetically, but affected oral and dental hygiene, kinaesthesia, feeding and speech to a marked degree. She was able to pronounce correctly most consonants and vowels in single words, but not at conversational levels of speed.

Moreover, she was subject to sudden and (to her parents) inexplicable pitch changes under stress; in the most unexpected circumstances she would loudly produce an unintelligible sentence in a deep rough voice. As she was both intelligent and well behaved, this peculiarity was very distressing to both parents and child.

Three days after surgery, all huskiness and involuntary pitch changes had disappeared, and speech in short utterances was clear. The patient became optimistic and eager to try her improved skills in speech; however, she still required therapy for a lisp and control of both articulation and salivation during connected utterance.

There were several examples of patients with anomalies of voice, including huskiness or hoarseness; a very loud, soft or weak voice; or an inability to vary the pitch, resulting in the patient talking only on a monotone. Many of these problems normalised spontaneously after successful surgery, without the need for therapy to be heavily focussed on these symptoms. Articulation problems, however, required very direct work.

LOWERED SELF ESTEEM

Although relatively little mention of tongue tie exists in the literature, it is interesting to note that of the case histories quoted, many imply lowered self-esteem and negative responses to the condition. Oldfield describes a typical case as follows:

> A young man aged 22 came to me because he was tongue tied ... I freed his tongue and his disability disappeared. If his short frenum had been divided when he was a baby, he could have been saved unnecessary embarrassment at school, and in his work afterwards. The fact that he found this deformity troublesome should be a guide to parents and help them to decide that a small operation is necessary, although disability may not be apparent in a small baby, unless it has had feeding difficulties.[2]

Self image

I observed during my study that children reacted to the frustrations of tongue tie with behavioural problems that reflected the organic problem: messy table manners, slow eating habits, fussiness over textures of food, persistent dribbliness or 'splashing' when talking vehemently. These symptoms are socially unacceptable and determine the way the child is seen by parents and contemporaries. They affect the self-image of the patient.

From an early age these children have been aware of having failed at eating fast, licking an ice cream, sticking their tongues out for the doctor, and talking properly. When dribbling persists it arouses strong negative reactions from people around them. Relatives are less likely to be warmly demonstrative towards a dribbly child.

I have also seen very depressed children, who have reacted to criticism as rejection; they have responded with sadness, 'laziness', eye blinking, twitching and complaints of pain. More assertive or very intelligent children develop masking behaviour, such as talking through clenched teeth or in a monotone, reducing the length of their utterances or manipulating the adult into doing most of the talking.

Despite the myth that surgery is only justified in cases of tongue tie when children have signifi-
cant disturbances of feeding and speech, many children with those very difficulties continue to suffer the limitations of their condition without the benefit of surgery. Instead, prolonged speech therapy is instituted, and improvement—if it occurs—is very slow.

Cecil, a 7-year-old boy, was seen for assessment only. There was a known history of tongue tie in at least two family members, and feeding in infancy was marred by choking and aspiration of milk until he was 18 months old. Chewing solids was not mastered until he was 2 years and 6 months old. Consequently, breastfeeding was continued until this time. When assessed, he still preferred to eat soft foods, and could not lick.

Cecil's tongue tie extended to the lingual margin and was easily seen. It travelled across the buccal floor in a fan shape, ending at the base of the incisors. Food stuck constantly to the child's teeth, lips and hard palate, and had to be extracted manually. As a small child he had dribbled profusely, and he now had extensive dental caries. Lingual activity and oral kinaesthesia were both poor, and although he had corrected various articulatory errors with speech therapy, no learned posture could be maintained for more than a few seconds. Thus, speech was almost unintelligible, and he spoke in a soft mumble with his mouth half closed.

These problems were of great significance for Cecil and his family. The child felt vulnerable and was shy of exposing his difficulties. His weaknesses had forced him into a position of dependancy, which had in turn fostered emotional immaturity. His mother was constantly on duty, interpreting for him when he did speak, and intervening to protect him from embarrassment. He was so sensitive about his failings that he performed assessment tasks with his eyes shut, to avoid seeing the reactions of the listener. This 7-year-old's confidence and self esteem were both very low, and it is not hard to imagine his probable difficulties at school.

Cecil was a good example of the toll the hidden agenda of tongue tie takes of its sufferers.

Behaviour

Children have been observed to react to the frustrations of limited tongue movement with anger, shyness or sadness. Insightful parents are quick to recognise signs of disquiet in their children. I have often been told that toddlers of 12 and 18 months are aware that they cannot perform lingual movements and have observed that they display some concern or sadness when asked to indulge in such activity. However supportive the environment, children will produce individual, unique and unpredictable reactions to limitations of lingual function.

One 2-year-old I saw was the only son of young and inexperienced parents. Little Peter was quickly categorised as an unusually troublesome member of the 'terrible two' brigade, and figured in a television programme under that title where he was seen flinging blocks and throwing a temper–tantrum. He also had a very tight tongue tie. After surgery, and some counselling sessions in which it was made clear to his mother that the aetiology of his 'terribleness' was rooted in frustration, Peter calmed down. His behaviour changed both in the sessions and at home. Concentration span and language improved, and he would sit and listen to stories and ask questions. Changes were more easily effected because Peter was under 3 years, he had a good surgical result and his family was willing to implement the changes in management that were recommended.

Manifestations of anger

It is important to realise that the speech pathologist will often see some very angry children who cannot let go of symptoms forced on them by their limited tongue movements. These will have been reinforced by environmental reaction, so that the behaviour pattern remains long after the cause of the problems was removed by surgery, however successful.

Eating habits

Messy table manners, persistent dribbling and dependency are frequent complaints that parents make of the child with tongue tie. Particularly in families where neat eating habits are valued, the one who has a tongue tie becomes a target of criticism, and children are aware that they are being labelled as naughty, sulky, messy eaters, lazy speakers and fussy feeders.

From an early age these children have been aware of having failed at eating fast, licking an ice cream, sticking their tongues out for the doctor, and talking properly. When dribbling persists it arouses strong negative reactions from people around them. Relatives are much less likely to be warmly demonstrative to a dribbly child.

Many children whose tongue tie prevents them from clearing food off their teeth resort to removing shreds of food from the cheek pouches with a hooked finger—an unsightly business, sure to bring down the wrath of parents and elders on the child's head! Unfortunately, such tricks are also very habit forming and become the nucleus of a cluster of anti-social eating behaviours if they persist. Some mothers of children in the study said they were forced to feed their messy eaters separately.

In one case, the sibling with tongue tie was the child of a previous spouse and very quickly became a scapegoat. Although his surgery was successful, he needed play therapy and counselling before he could relinquish his irritating passive–aggressive eating habits. Unfortunately his very real symptoms had given him a chance of enjoying individual attention and although this was negative attention, he was unwilling to forfeit it by conforming. Symptom formation is always a possibility when children have to cope with physical difficulties that have socially unacceptable consequences.

One 3-year-old had a very poor feeding history and, when seen, had developed a head banging habit which was indulged in seven or eight times a day. This reduced slightly when therapy began. After surgery he put on weight rapidly and the head banging ceased even before there was any improvement in communication skills.

Parental reactions

Parents can exhibit a wide variety of reactions to their children's problems.

The boy described below did not receive any therapy, had surgery late and was expected to improve without guidance during his vulnerable teenage years:

> At the age of 14 a dentist's son was referred on account of a tongue tie which hindered tongue movement when he played his clarinet. Examination revealed a definite tongue tie in an otherwise normal boy. The tie was successfully divided, but the father wrote 6 weeks later: "As he is at the best of times a careless speaker, it is difficult to say that there has been much improvement in his speech".[19]

Parents who have tongue tie themselves or have had relatives with tongue tie were in a sensitive situation—guilt was aroused at having passed down a problem requiring surgery to a beloved child. If the parent had suffered with a tongue tie, some envy might be shown of a child who was fortunate enough to be diagnosed. Unless such feelings are acknowledged, or verbalised tactfully by the speech pathologist, the child can be burdened with over-critical correction and counterproductive moralisations, so that the therapy is overtly or covertly sabotaged.

Infant reactions

One child aged 10 months was seen who had not mastered tongue retraction when accepting a piece of biscuit. He was very hungry, but in reaching for the biscuit his tongue thrusted and pushed the biscuit out. Eventually his mother had to help him by pushing the biscuit in and shutting his lips with her fingers so as to avert a tantrum.

Young and inexperienced mothers would undoubtedly be as frustrated as their babies if often faced with such apparently 'contrary behaviour' during feeding.

The youngest children referred to me with tongue tie showed clearly their awareness of their particular difficulties. Philip, aged 12 months, would refuse to attempt to mimic facial grimaces if a tongue thrusting movement was demanded. A week after surgery, he was seen looking at himself in the mirror and poking his tongue out, then calling to his mother and poking his tongue out at her.

Bruce, aged 9 months, was clingy and dependent, and often had to be rescued from the robust play of peers at playgroup. A fortnight after surgery, his babbling developed into single words, and he began to stamp his feet and say 'no' to assertive playmates. He also began, for the first time, to explore his mouth with his fingers.

When these facts are assembled in a case history, their impact is unquestionable. As speech pathologists, teachers, doctors or parents, we ask ourselves why such painful disabilities are allowed to remain when they can be overcome so easily. Is it because children cannot complain about their difficulties in the way that adults can, and do?

Perhaps the answer lies in the fact that all the relevant data need to be recognised and put together before their importance can be acknowledged and appropriate action taken.

4 Assessment Criteria

Since tongue tie has not been considered to be a cause of serious speech difficulties, there has been no methodology in the field of speech pathology for assessment of the condition.

During the course of the study and in order to determine whether a patient's tongue tie warranted surgical intervention, I developed a Tongue tie Assessment Protocol (TAP) which was based on seven important criteria:

1. Cosmetic appearance
2. Oral hygiene and dental health
3. Feeding skills
4. Lingual movement
5. Oral kinaesthesia
6. Speech
7. Emotional status

The importance of taking account of factors other than simply physical appearance and speech was pointed out by Young and Sacks after their 1978 study in Philadelphia. They concluded that any evaluation for ankyloglossia must include 'assessment of vegetative function [of the tongue], dental status and speech production ...'[28] These three aspects are incorporated in the seven criteria detailed above.

Detailed instructions for conducting a tongue tie assessment using TAP are given in Appendix B. The TAP requires that a score of 0 to 4 be given for each of the seven criteria, depending on the degree of variation from normal noted. The scores for each criteria are then added to obtain the total score. If the total score is 15 or less, a conclusion can be made that surgical release is warranted.

While stressing that each case must be decided on its merits, surgery is not recommended for children with global developmental delay or multiple handicaps unless the patient is judged to be capable of benefitting from an improved degree of lingual mobility. (An example of one happy exception to this is described in Chapter 7, Case History 8.)

DEVISING ASSESSMENT MEASURES

In 1968, Fletcher and Meldrum successfully used a modified boley gauge with measuring callipers and a linear scale to measure sublingual dimensions in 210 students whose mean age was 11.5 years;[10] and in 1985 Williams and Waldron used acrylic blocks of increasing thickness to measure jaw opening, and a standard machinist's calliper to measure tongue elevation.[8]

However, it is felt that such methods suffer from complex technology. While mechanical measurements of the tongue and its capacities are relevant in research, they would be perceived by patients as intrusive acts which would, in the long run, be counter-productive in therapy.

Since tongue movements tend to be fluid, and subjects with tongue tie lack the control to hold and maintain a position unaided, the task of assessing movements for the purpose of the study seemed almost impossible. It was difficult to find an acceptable way of correlating the sounds made in speech with the position or shape of the individual tongue in the oral space.

As described by Fletcher and Meldrum:

> … simply looking in the mouth and making an impressionistic judgement is likely to be heavily biased by such factors as size and configuration of the oral cavity, absolute and relative size of the entire corpus of the tongue, posture of the tongue within the oral cavity, and discrepancies in speech articulation.'[10]

Fletcher and Meldrum also found that 'less restriction of the anterior part of the tongue by the lingual frenulum is associated with fewer errors in speech articulation performance.[10]

They also comment that:

> West, Ansberry, and Carr (pp. 179–180) repudiate the effects of ankyloglossia on speech with the assertion that this condition "can have very little adverse effect upon production of speech sounds." They advance the equally non-tested alternative postulation that "agenesis of the tongue tip" accounts for many defects in speech articulation which are erroneously attributed to ankyloglossia.[10]

There were only two instances found in the literature of the speech of patients with tongue tie being compared with the speech of those without a tie. Fletcher and Meldrum assessed 40 children in the same age group, divided into two sets on the basis of relative length of lingual frenum. They found that '… 20 subjects with limited lingual freedom made a total of 60 errors in speech articulation in contrast with eight such errors by subjects with greater lingual freedom.'[10]

Williams and Waldron[8] in their article on 'Assessment of lingual function when ankyloglossia (tongue-tie) is suspected', used:

- Linear measurement of the lingual frenum (from sublingual gland to lingual

insertion), and linear measurement of tongue tip (from lingual frenular attachment to the tongue tip).
- Timed rapid repetitive lingual movements (after Fletcher) and a speech articulation test, to screen the accuracy of tongue-tip sounds.

They felt that the patient who could produce tongue-tip sounds accurately would not be a candidate for surgery. However, my experience suggests that all speech sounds need to be considered equally, both in words and sentences, and also at speed, to ensure that results obtained are accurate. The diadochokinetic test should always carry greater weight than a test of articulation.

In the literature there has often been an emphasis placed on tongue-tip sounds, as being particularly at risk in cases of speech difficulty. Block upheld this traditional theory about articulatory errors: 'When there is a tongue tie, the sounds that may be affected are tongue tip sounds such as T, D, N, L, SH, S, ZH, R, Z, TH.'[17]

The sounds made by the tongue tip are so conspicuous by their absence in so-called 'severe' or 'true' cases of tongue tie that in the past some authorities have preferred the notion of agenesis of the tongue tip to an aetiology of tongue tie!

However, the study showed great variety in the types of error, and that lateralisation of consonants is also common. Where the 'tip' of the tongue is anchored, the sides of the tongue become visibly over-active such that air is directed laterally, causing a preponderance of distorted or lateralised consonants.

OBJECTIVES OF ASSESSMENT

Devising an assessment process which would be practical, relevant to practising speech pathologists, speedy to perform and yet equally applicable to babies, older children and adults, was thus a challenging task.

The objectives of assessment were to ascertain:
- whether tongue tie existed;
- if it existed, to what degree it incapacitated the individual;
- whether surgical release is likely to make a significant difference; and
- what contribution could be expected from speech therapy.

It was not practical to have a control group for the purpose of research since this would have been composed, perforce, of those patients who were on a long waiting list for therapy or surgery. Patients presenting with tongue tie were suffering from a variety of symptoms and were not favourably disposed toward the idea of being in a control group.

The assessment, therefore, needed to provide ongoing measurement of the symptoms of tongue tie, the effects of the symptoms on the functioning of the patient, and the rate of progress after surgery. Since there was no existing measure of standard tongue lengths, movements, or lingual size or shape that was capable of being applied to the age range of patients being studied (9 months to adults), the task of devising an assessment procedure was very challenging.

THE METHOD DEVISED

The assessment process finally devised (the TAP) is applicable to all patients, but in the case of babies who are not yet speaking, it has, of necessity, been simplified. Not all babies will be at the same developmental level, hence it is important that therapeutic insight into babies' facial play is used when selecting tasks.

Infants need to be old enough, if they are expected to be able to imitate tongue protrusion or licking or sound production as requested. Infants under 6 months are therefore assessed only on feeding history, inspection, and digital palpation of the tie. For the purposes of therapy rather than research, variation in the tasks set is of course acceptable, as long as goals are age-appropriate.

Although the subjective nature of the assessment may be a criticism of this method, familiarity with the problems which obtain in patients with tongue tie is of course an advantage during assessment, and can counter-balance subjectivity. Subjective clinical judgements of quality, clumsiness or anxiety will always need to be made by speech pathologists. Exposure to numbers of such patients should help solve this problem. It is hoped that the TAP will give speech pathologists a basis for confidence in their assessments.

CASE HISTORY

The taking of a detailed case history is seen as a vital ingredient of the assessment process. Without sufficient background information a differential diagnosis cannot be carried out. For instance, if the patient had been slow in developing all skills, poor feeding and oral co-ordination would have been part of a global picture rather than a direct consequence of the tie. Mild cerebral palsy could cause poor control of salivation, and environmental deprivation could relate to poor oral hygiene. Emotional problems or poor mother–infant bonding could also affect feeding.

A detailed case history can provide information of a family history of tongue tie, which in fact was present in a number of the cases studied. Frequently, those patients who had a family history of tongue tie had a greater degree of disability and showed involvement in most of the areas I eventually considered as criteria for the diagnosis of tongue tie.

Very often, taking a detailed case history and asking the right questions will trigger parental recollections of events which are most relevant to the diagnosis, but which have not been kept in mind because they are considered to be no longer of immediate significance. This particularly applies to details concerning breastfeeding, where the mother is only too happy to forget her past discomforts and disappointments with an experience she may have been eagerly anticipating. Open discussion of the difficulties can also serve to dissipate the guilt that the mother may have been harbouring about her inability to feed the baby well.

As in the case of other patients with speech defects, the whole child in his or her environment must be considered, and the taking of a comprehensive history is a vital part of the diagnostic process.

IMPORTANCE OF VISUAL ASSESSMENT

Prior to conducting an assessment it is extremely important that the frenum is inspected and any abnormality is observed. In order to make an accurate judgement in this regard the practitioner must be familiar with the different appearances of the frenum in a wide spectrum of cases embracing patients of all ages and various degrees of severity. Many different ties are illustrated in the colour plates obtained during the study and included in this publication.

In babies, who are usually referred specifically because of feeding difficulty, a visual evaluation may establish the following:

- the tongue may move very little;
- the tip of the tongue may be pulled under on mild extension;
- the anterior part of the tongue may be heart-shaped; and
- the frenum feels tight on palpation.

This information, with a careful history of breastfeeding, bottle feeding and reaction to introduction of solids, is usually sufficient for diagnosis of tongue tie in very small babies.

The diagnosis of tongue tie in babies relies as heavily on seeing the under-surface of the tongue as on a history of feeding difficulty. Unfortunately, visual assessment of that part of the tongue in

babies is often difficult. Coupled with the general lack of information regarding the effects of tongue tie, this difficulty may be implicated in late diagnosis of the condition.

Once ankyloglossia, or tongue tie, is accepted as a condition suitably treated by surgical intervention, the diagnosis in babies should be simplified, as it should be acceptable for the practitioner to diagnose immediately after observing the tie. However, older patients who have escaped diagnosis at an early age, for one reason or another, will obviously need a full assessment for differential diagnosis.

In older patients, it is possible that a diagnosis of dyspraxia may be mistakenly made by speech pathologists unfamiliar with tongue tie. However, once the tie has been seen and identified, we may be prepared for those equivocal signs that simulate dyspraxia. Patients with tongue tie will show an absence of current neurological pathology, or a history indicating previous neurological dysfunction. 'Normal' tongue movements will not occur involuntarily, when they cannot be performed on command, as will happen in the case of a dyspraxic patient. Further, in dyspraxic patients, the lips are involved as readily as the tongue, while with the patient with tongue tie, lip movement will be generally better than tongue movement.

THE SEVEN CRITERIA

The following seven criteria form the basis for assessment of tongue tie using the TAP. They were selected because they were consistently found to be affected in the majority of subjects with tongue tie and, in my experience, are generally found to be within normal limits in patients without tongue tie.

1. Cosmetic appearance

The tongue is capable of subtle changes of shape and size. It has been described as being: '... completely a soft tissue structure with no non-mobile landmarks.'[10]

Professor Barclay gives a good description of the difference between a normal frenum and an abnormal frenum leading to tongue tie:

> The normal lingual fraenum, located on the ventral surface of the mouth, consists of little more than a band of connective tissue covered by a thin layer of mucous membrane. In the condition of tongue-tie, or ankyloglossia, a well developed fraenum may come as far forward as the tip of the tongue above, and the lingual aspect of the mandible below. Some abnormal lingual fraenae contain dense fibrous connective tissue, and occasionally include a few fibres of the genioglossus muscle.[21]

During my study, certain appearances of the tongue, and certain mannerisms which appeared to aid in the performance of assessment tasks, became very familiar. The appearance of the tongue at rest (including its size, shape and accustomed position), as well as its appearance during activities such as speech, yawning and feeding was nearly always noted as different (see Plate 1).

The indentation or notching of the anterior margin of the tongue was seen on almost all subjects with tongue tie. This notching of the tongue is permanent (see Plate 2) and frequently continues to be seen even in those subjects who have undergone surgery in infancy. The apparent absence of the tongue tip is frequently observed (see Plate 3). However, the presence of the tongue tip together with a prominent, short or tight frenum (see Plate 4) suggests a 'mild' tie, and is therefore a relevant feature to note.

The frenum itself can vary from a thin transparent membrane (see Plate 5) to a short thick tie (see Plate 6). There is frequently variation also in the extent of the tie. Some ties commence just behind the lower front teeth (see Plate 7), while others are deeply embedded under the tongue (see Plate 8).

Some ties extend right up to the tongue tip, even pulling the tip of the tongue downward (see Plate 9). Other ties are very short, so that the tongue is not able to stretch far in any direction (see Plate 10), and three ties were seen during the study which were so short that it was almost impossible to raise the tongue to view the tie! The tongue, therefore, had the appearance of being fused to the floor of the mouth. Some text books discriminate between partial and complete ankyloglossia—a tongue fused to the buccal floor being classified as complete ankyloglossia.

Most ties are easily visible or can be inferred from typical movements performed. Some ties may be seen to extend across the floor of the mouth and spread into a fan shape at the base of the lower incisors (see Plate 11). While many tongues are large, thick and immobile looking, others may look small and ineffective.

Two descriptions of the appearance of the tongue that is affected by tongue tie are given below:

> The tongue is tied down by an abnormally tight lingual frenulum which may be fibrous or muscular.[26]

> ... the frenum of the tongue is short with a thin mucous membrane attachment in some cases, and a thick fibrosed attachment in others, depending upon the extent of involvement of the genioglossus muscle ... The forward extension of the tongue is restricted, and shows notching at the midline ... the tongue frequently will not elevate ... In forward extension, the tongue displays a curling movement and the posterior margins of the tongue become wide and bulky.[3]

In milder cases of tongue tie, the tongue is frequently long, large and capable of forceful thrusting, but quite uncontrolled in movement. The tie can be clearly seen as a thick white column of tissue. Although such variation in appearance occurs, other observed signs may soon be identified as typical and are not found in subjects without a tongue tie.

The point of insertion of the frenum also makes a characteristic circular depression towards the middle of the tongue. This was observed during the study in most patients while speaking and when attempting to elevate the tongue (see Plate 2).

Interestingly, this depression may also be seen in very young babies whose tongues are capable of feeding and pre-speech movements only but who do not have tongue ties. It is also seen in some children whose lingual movements are very clumsy and who display severe articulatory defects.

Whitman and Rankow describe the circular depression seen in patients with tongue tie thus:

> ... the tip comes straight up, while the dorsum remains flat, in fact there is a dimpling in the dorsal area which corresponds to the insertion of the restraining genioglossus muscle.[26]

In babies with tongue tie, the short membrane may be attached to the tongue tip, which is notched and turns under. There is poverty of lingual movement, with no protrusion beyond the lower lip or elevation to the upper lip. If the tongue protrudes beyond the lower lip, it may be pulled downward by the tightness of the frenum. Dribbling is often profuse, even when the baby is not teething.

If the patients with blunt-ended tongues seen in my study actually had an agenesis of the tongue tip, it would be difficult to explain why there should have been a gradual 'genesis', or appearance, of the tongue tip after surgery and the assiduous practice of the exercises prescribed! It should be stressed, perhaps, that this alteration in the shape of the tongue did not occur in cases where specified tongue pointing exercises had not been carried out for a sufficient period of time.

2. Oral hygiene and dental health

Poor oral hygiene, having both social and medical ramifications, is a most significant but little known consequence of tongue tie.

Signs such as dribbling, apparent hypersalivation during speech in older patients, involuntary splashing of saliva, the presence of food debris around the mouth or stuck on the hard palate and teeth after a meal, rashes around the mouth (see Plate 12) and dental caries (see Plates 6 and 10) can all be consequences of tongue tie.

Dental malocclusions, irregular eruption of teeth and open bite are often associated with tongue tie (see Plate 13). It was noted during the study that dental caries were found in many of the children who were over the age of seven. In some cases these children were from families where the level of dental hygiene was very good and the child with tongue tie was the only child in the family who had caries.

3. Feeding skills

When infants were seen during the study, a comprehensive feeding history was taken. Breastfeeding may have been associated with problems ranging from sore or bleeding nipples in the mother to failure to thrive in the infant. It was important, therefore, to understand what had happened, and guide the parent toward seeing the problems as they really were.

Observation of feeding of infants with tongue tie may reveal difficulties, such as dribbling of milk while sucking, slow feeding because of ineffective sucking, frequent loss of suction and a clicking noise which accompanies it.

One infant seen had such poor swallowing that milk leaked intermittently from the nostrils while drinking. Some babies would feed better on one breast than on the other, and the clicking sound would only be heard on the 'difficult' breast.

Feeding problems, once thought to be major predictors of the validity of tongue tie, are not always simple to assess. Often the problem has been overcome or ameliorated by the time the patient is seen. Relieved parents tend to concentrate on the present, and stress that the child is 'better now'.

However, careful questioning and the taking of a very detailed case history can reveal facts that have been forgotten. Where the problem has persisted, it can become involved with behaviour and will often be seen as naughtiness or helplessness.

Conversely, some 'good' children with highly conscientious mothers will not be seen as having difficulty, although allowances and adjustments are constantly being made to facilitate feeding: vegetables being blended, drinking water throughout the meal being excused as necessary (even when the quantity is inappropriate), and the swallowing of large unchewed lumps is described as 'eating well'.

Adult patients, being more in control of their lifestyles than children, may feel entitled to pursue their preference for food that is readily masticated, and can choose to eat finely cut-up Chinese or Italian food and to drink as desired while eating their meals.

4. Lingual movement

Anomalies of Movement

There are many anomalies of lingual movement which may be recognised instantly in patients with tongue tie. Common movements of the tongue observed during the study could be described as sluggish, uncontrolled, jerky, unusual, overactive or underactive.

The often conspicuous nature of the condition is striking. Bizarre movements of a characteristic nature are frequently seen in the tongue during activities such as attempts at lateral licking (*see*

Plate 14) or attempts at protrusion (*see Plate 15)* and often make the tie very obvious.

The enforced curtailment of movement in the tongue sometimes engenders a frantic lingual restlessness, which can easily be observed in patients with a mild tongue tie.

The sides of the tongue are very active (*see Plate 16)*, they heave and bulge, and the young child might be seen enjoying this unattractive activity. Although the limitation of movement may be categorised as 'mild', these cases often demonstrate very severe long-term detrimental effects both physiologically and emotionally. (An example of such a case is described in Chapter 7, Case History 2.)

In patients with a more severe tongue tie, movement is obviously limited; however, it can still be very forceful. In these cases, strange rolling and twisting movements take place during attempts to touch or locate parts of the mouth, and are therefore often seen during assessment while speaking rather than at rest. An attempt at downward pointing is shown in Plate 17, where direction is skewed, and often both notching and medial lingual grooving are seen.

Movement in young babies can be assessed digitally, by inserting a finger in the mouth with the nail down and the finger tip near the soft palate. While a normal tongue will begin sucking movements which 'cup' the tongue and produce a wavelike motion along the whole finger, the baby with tongue tie may just tap the finger upward. The frenulum will feel tight to the touch, and the back of the tongue will be seen to rise although the tongue is anchored at the front.

Limitations of Movement

Initially in the study it was very difficult to assess and record limitations of movement. Even with the gross limitation of movement suffered by many subjects with tongue tie, the tongue would change its appearance so much during observation that it was difficult to be satisfied with the assessment.

Eventually I decided to consider the success or failure to achieve six arbitrarily chosen 'standard tongue positions', which were:

- protrusion with downward pointing;
- horizontal pointing;
- protrusion with upward pointing;
- circumlocution;
- lateral movement; and
- retraction of the tongue.

All these positions are commonly used during everyday functioning, such as licking, protruding the tongue, performing what dentists refer to as 'internal oral toilet', yawning or pointing the tongue in a desired direction.

For purposes of comparison, adults and children over the age of three without tongue tie were asked to perform these movements; not surprisingly, they were all able to do so. For the purpose of accuracy, subjects of the study were photographed attempting the movements pre and post-operatively. This subsequently proved to be a most significant and useful measure.

• *Protrusion with downward pointing:* Nearly all subjects with tongue tie could extend the tongue for a considerable distance downwards. Examination by demanding a non-specific 'stick out your tongue' is therefore bound to be misleading when used to diagnose tongue tie *(see Plate 17).*

• *Horizontal pointing:* This presents problems for the patient with a tongue tie. Often the tongue will not protrude beyond the vermilion, or when it can do so, cannot remain steady. The strongest pull on the tongue tip seems to be in this position *(see Plate 15).* This difficulty is well described by Ketty and Sciullo:

The forward extension of the tongue is restricted and shows notching at the midline. In some cases, the tongue, in forward extension, does not reach the vermilion border of the lip; it rests in the mucobuccal fold. In other cases, the tongue in over-extension may reach the vermilion border but the tip of the tongue is forced downwards.[3]

• *Protrusion with upward pointing:* This position is almost always impossible for the patient with tongue tie to achieve. Often there is no understanding of how to attempt the task. If a mirror is provided, children who have previously had speech therapy will attempt to support the tongue on the lower lip and thereby to raise the tongue. Strong extraneous movements of the head (tilting upwards), lower jaw (protruding and pushing up), and eyes (rolling up), will be used to assist in the effort.

A few patients can protrude and touch the top lip while the lips are shut and the jaws grip the tongue *(see Plate 4),* but are unable to elevate with relaxed or parted lips. Upward curling of the sides of the tongue *(see Plate 3)* is often seen in patients with tongue tie. Often patients will ask how this movement should be performed. If the tie is mild, the tongue might be elevated involuntarily outside the mouth but not intra-orally, and the movement will usually not be performed consistently.

One patient seen during the study had a long history of previous speech therapy (five speech pathologists!) and could achieve elevation while looking in a mirror, concentrating, and slowly raising the tongue with the aid of the lower lip. Speech therapy had given him understanding of the task but not the ability to perform it freely.

Ketty and Sciullo describe the inability of these patients to elevate their tongues thus:

When requested to touch the roof of the mouth with the mouth open, the tongue frequently will not elevate. If the tongue elevates, the anterior dorsal surface of the tip of the tongue is pulled backwards onto the ventral surface with a downward pull of the tongue.[3]

Certain authorities feel that this problem can also cause swallowing difficulties. Tuerk and Lubit maintain that ankyloglossia resulting in the inability to raise the tongue to the roof of the palate may prevent development of the normal adult swallow pattern. This in turn results in a continuation of the infantile swallow and subsequently leads to an open bite malocclusion.[31]

Many of the children, and all of the adults seen, swallowed with the tongue pushing against the front teeth.

• *Circumlocution:* The patient is asked to lick around the mouth in a circular movement. Many patients use a hasty lateral rubbing of the lower lip with the under-side of the tongue, and do not attempt to lick around the top lip. Some use the middle (blade) of the tongue and rub it along the top lip. Some use the lower lip in a lateral rubbing movement. This movement is of course significant for social reasons and for oral hygiene.

• *Lateral Movements:* The subject is asked to move the tongue slowly, then quickly, from the left to the right hand corner of the lips. First, the inside corners of the lips are aimed for, then the outside corners. The patient is thus asked to discriminate between inside *(see Plate 18)* and outside *(see Plate 19)*, left and right, fast and slow. Small children who have not as yet mastered right/left identification can be asked to go from 'this side to that'.

Great variety in results is possible here, with some patients finding this task very hard to do. Being entirely visible, this exercise can be mastered with practice, and is a useful therapeutic tool.

• *Retraction of the Tongue:* This was also found to be a useful movement to observe. Many patients

have little or no idea of the depth of the oral space and cannot imagine pushing the tongue backwards. Retraction of the tongue allows the tie to be seen *(see Plate 20)* even without an intentional movement from the patient. It is often possible to elicit this movement from young subjects during yawning or loud crying.

5. Oral kinaesthesia
It is necessary to have an idea of the patient's ability to visualise the oral space; to initiate and to copy movements at slow, moderate and fast rates; and to compare this with the patient's ability to perform the same tasks when aided by visual clues.

A mirror, or the speech pathologist's face (seen full face and sideways performing the task), or a photograph provide adequate clues. When toddlers are being assessed, they are asked to copy grimaces or sounds, slowly, then faster. When assessing babies for the purpose of diagnosis, it is more practical to get a good look at the tie, rather than to attempt to assess their level of oral kinaesthetic ability.

Older children may have the task described to them, then be asked to copy it with or without the mirror. Adults would also be asked to describe verbally how they performed certain tasks involving oromuscular manipulation. Often patients with tongue tie are unable to discriminate between labial, lingual and palatal contacts without visual clues *(see Plate 21)*.

6. Speech
Speech problems are not always mentioned by patients or their parents seeking help because of a tongue tie. It was clearly seen during the study that intelligent patients were able to adopt masking strategies in order to hide the symptom or to distract the listener.

Patients may have learnt that talking slowly, quietly, in a monotone, in short sentences or with the mouth nearly shut, permits them to enunciate clearly enough for speech to pass muster. Careful investigation can unmask problems. Frequently, nonverbal aspects of communication are also affected, including flexibility of pitch, rhythm, volume and variations of facial expression.

Often the speech has been adequate for immature stages of language development but has proved to be inadequate for more adult or mature communication. The speech pathologist may be told a story of normal speech that is deteriorating and be misled into seeing the problem as solely behavioural.

Sifting of the information received will show that speech only appeared to be normal because of the small demands made on the patient at earlier developmental levels. Speech assessment must include testing the ability of the patient to speak clearly in connected speech; with lengthy utterances; and with changes of speed, pitch and volume. Voice quality must also be checked, since these patients often show a tendency to become dysphonic or excessively nasal under stress.

A striking finding in the study was that, contrary to popular opinion, the lingual sounds were not the only, or even the primary, sounds to be defective in the speech of patients with tongue tie. Very often sounds that were quite clear in isolation or even in single words were produced incorrectly in sentences, or 'connected' speech.

Where specific sounds are consistently defective, lingual sounds are as likely to be affected as any other. Tongue thrusting on sibilants is often present—which was an unexpected finding of the study. In fact, such thrusting is highly consistent with the disability. It is due to an inability to control and grade the tongue movement that shapes the S. Compounding the difficulty, the shape of the tongue in a patient with tongue tie is unusually broad and flat, and often dented along the margin in the midline.

It might be mentioned here that the kindergarten teacher of a patient attending for a post-operative follow-up appointment in the course of the study, volunteered the information that she too had a tongue tie. She found it hard to talk clearly when tired, and had a tongue-thrust swallow. A parent with a tongue tie revealed that he consciously pronounced the L sound by 'sucking on the palate'. These are examples of strategies adopted by adult patients with unrepaired tongue ties which remain hidden, appearing only as idiosyncratic behaviour.

7. Emotional status

The purpose of including this aspect of the patient in assessment is twofold. Firstly, to determine how much of an impact the tongue tie has on the patient's self esteem. Secondly, to allow the speech pathologist a fuller appreciation of the patient's difficulties. Observed personality traits offer clues, which when noted with relevant history can explain a patient's timidity, hostility or reluctance in the session.

It is reasonable to assume that experiences of failure, frustration or rejection because of clumsiness or ugliness produce trauma in both adults and children. We accept the emotional consequences of cleft lip or cerebral palsy, as we do those of milder speech problems, but it is not commonly realised that the patient with ankyloglossia also suffers (see Plate 22).

Ketty and Sciullo describe a case of ankyloglossia with psychological implications[3]. After consultation with a speech pathologist, they performed surgery on a boy who was 4 years and 6 months old, because of ankyloglossia, incipient dental caries, emotional disturbances and speech defects. The father insisted on the operation for 'sexual reasons', presumably to ensure the ability to kiss normally. This was a concern that some parents in my study also displayed.

When the situation of the patient with tongue tie has been compounded by the birth of siblings, illness, feeding problems and communication difficulty, there are pronounced effects on the family. One parent of a baby with tongue tie, who had tongue tie himself, recalled feelings as an adolescent of anxiety and pain about his self-image and embarrassment about his oral hygiene.

It must also be realised that severe disturbance of feeding, particularly breastfeeding, will have an impact on mother–infant bonding, and may have behavioural repercussions, at least in the early years. How successfully these problems are resolved may determine future interactions. Where breastfeeding has been traumatic for the mother and child, most mothers react with guilt and self-blame. Some mothers will reject the infant who bites the breast, but it is also possible that the infant will be left hungry and frustrated and hence very angry with the mother.

For one patient in the study, the severity of his emotional problems prompted the decision to postpone surgical intervention in favour of more urgent priorities. Mike, aged 6 years, was a severely infantilised boy with a moderate degree of tongue tie. Saliva poured continually from his open lips, and his speech was unclear and some-times nasal, but he had the ability to close the palatal sphincter in structured tasks. I felt he was a profoundly disturbed child, with remote affect, inability to play, autistic-type mannerisms, and an obsessive interest in computers. I recommended that he should have psychological counselling and make some improvement in his relationships before surgery was attempted.

Thorough assessment using the TAP, supplemented by the taking of a full case history, will often reveal hitherto unsuspected consequences of tongue tie in both adults and children. An important advantage of this protocol is the way it allows the speech pathologist and surgeon to understand that the consequences of this condition may warrant surgery even when the degree of physical limitation ensuing from the condition is apparently mild.

Often the assessment will show that the score on limitation of movement is relatively good in cases where prior speech therapy has been undertaken, but if the score for oral kinaesthesia is not acceptable, speech will be found to be poor. As the next chapter will show, assessment with the TAP prior to operation or therapy allows monitoring of progress by re-assessment on the same parameters after operation and therapy.

5 Surgery for Tongue Tie

The speech pathologist often experiences situations where tonsillectomy, removal of vocal nodules or cleft palate surgery have had to be recommended. However, in these cases the surgeon bears the responsibility of being the major decision maker.

In the case of tongue tie, speech pathologists are required to make very important judgements on the basis of function, and may not feel sufficiently experienced to advise. In view of past attitudes to surgery for tongue tie, they may be reluctant to express a controversial opinion. However, it is vitally important that the patient feels assured of the speech pathologist's confidence in the validity of any recommendations that are made.

CAN SURGERY HELP?

Surgical intervention is often not recommended because of a belief that it is only appropriate in very severe cases. Furthermore, for children over 3 years of age, surgery alone will not eliminate symptoms. It seems likely that the poor results of performing surgery with no follow-up speech therapy may have contributed to surgery being considered an ineffective and therefore inappropriate option.

Many children under 3 years do gradually develop normal oromuscular skills, including speech, once the tongue is adequately freed. It was found, however, that therapeutic supervision and guidance were advisable after operation for these young patients, for a period of 3 to 6 months, until they were seen to have acquired age-appropriate oromuscular function.

At present, as many patients are diagnosed late, a category of older patients remains, requiring both good surgery and task-specific speech therapy for effective management. Neither speech therapy, nor surgery alone, will remove the problems of the older patient.

In the case of infants with tongue tie, who are usually referred because of feeding difficulty, good surgery helps immediately. When the baby is put to the breast after frenulotomy, instant improvement in feeding is reported: the mother for the first time breastfeeds without suffering pain, and infant weight-gain is noted within the week. Most professionals today would agree that to deal with such a problem merely by putting the baby on a bottle is an unacceptable solution. However, many mothers are unwilling to admit their difficulties with breastfeeding; instead they see the problem as being due to their own inadequacy and manage the situation as best they can. In my experience, doctors are not always told of breastfeeding difficulties unless they are so major that the baby fails to thrive.

WHEN SURGERY IS RECOMMENDED

When discussing management with a parent whose child has been recommended for surgery, the speech pathologist needs to be knowledgable, empathetic and firm. Both patient and parents may have fears, reservations or questions that they are reluctant to reveal. On the other hand, they may be demanding and voluble in their requests for information, guarantees of success or predictions of future progress. Matters discussed should mirror the level of interest expressed, and it is important that the speech pathologist should not let preconceived notions of what is, or is not, of relevance to patients and parents dilute the potency of this very important interaction.

Children in particular will have difficulty in verbalising the exact nature of their fears about surgery. It should be remembered that many vital experiences of childhood which contribute to the most significant feelings and anxieties of children are below 'word level', and can only be demonstrated in play, or symptom formation. Overtly, children may deny fear, pain and reality—'I'm not afraid, it won't hurt', 'it will be good fun', 'I will have ice cream in hospital'—but if handled sensitively, they will reveal negative feelings of anxiety, insecurity, and anger.

Adult patients may doubt the efficacy of surgery for long-standing problems. However, as voluntary participants they tend to be highly motivated to cooperate in order to achieve maximum success.

Allowing and encouraging free verbalisation of feelings in parents and patients sets the scene for a trusting relationship between the care givers and the patient, and should make a considerable difference to the whole experience. Speech pathologists need to have an understanding of the facts and the dynamics of the situation and to control their own feelings of frustration or uncertainty.

Providing full information about the operation, including drawings and explanations, helps most parents to feel more comfortable. Being offered the opportunity to 'let off steam', to seek a second opinion or to express anxiety and uncertainty, allows the parent or patient to make decisions based on facts rather than on feelings.

CONFLICTING PRIORITIES
It must also be remembered that tongue tie is not confined to emotionally stable or well-adjusted subjects or families. As with any organic congenital condition, parents who are aggressive, rejecting or punitive, and siblings who are overprotective or competitive, may complicate the picture.

Sick parents or siblings may take attention away from the child with tongue tie whose operation may be postponed repeatedly on what seem to be minor grounds. Three children in the study did not have their surgery as recommended because a sibling had been diagnosed with cerebral palsy. Another child missed out on surgery because he had a cleft palate, upon which the parents blamed all the feeding problems.

Good therapeutic practice requires that speech pathologists use all their skills to bring reality to bear on the situation and to do this they must be well informed of the grounds for recommending surgery.

Where the tongue tie is part of a syndrome, other problems may appear to be more important because of their more drastic or life-threatening qualities.

During the study, tongue tie was found occurring in conjunction with hearing loss, developmental delay, hyperplasia of the dentine, cerebral palsy, haemophilia, cleft lip and palate, ear tags and cysts on the frenum lingua! The speech pathologist must be flexible enough to exercise understanding about parental priorities and be aware of reservations that families may have regarding surgery.

While it is our responsibility to see that parents have enough information to make an informed decision, making that decision is their prerogative. The wisdom of such a standpoint can be easily understood if we reflect that strong persuasion can seem to convince persons who are not assertive enough to disagree with the speech pathologist, but who may then choose not to follow through with plans and arrangements that are made, or to be so uncooperative that they effectively sabotage subsequent proceedings.

THE OPERATION THEN AND NOW

Tongue-tie surgery has been—and still is—performed in a variety of ways. New-born babies who have been identified as having tongue tie may have the thin membrane separated or torn by the midwife or obstetrician.

Less frequently, a doctor may perform the 'operation' in his surgery, seeing it as a minor procedure. However, the pain of the procedure, the difficulty of accurate division in the conscious patient and the risk of bleeding all make this an inappropriate approach.

Antony Wallace in 1963 had this to say about such 'snipping':

> Snipping of a tongue tie is unreservedly condemned. It is performed without anaesthesia … No sutures are used. This operation may be ineffective and, since it leaves two adjacent raw surfaces, the tie sometimes recurs. The profunda linguae veins, lingual arteries, and genioglossi have been "snipped" in error along with the frenulum, producing haemorrhage and suffocation.[19]

Sometimes the operation is seen as so simple, that it is performed with only a local anaesthetic. It is to be hoped that the following experience of one child I assessed is not a common one:

Jacob, aged three, had a severe degree of tongue tie, and was reported to have been operated on by a witch doctor! (This was evidently quite possible, as the hospital interpreter vouched for it.) Poor Jacob, fully conscious and protesting wildly, had his frenum clipped by the witch doctor in the presence of his father. An assistant had urged his principal to 'cut more, cut more', but Jacob protested so much that this was not done.

The incision was insufficient, but the task of clipping the tongue of a screaming, bleeding, terrified child might be expected to shake the nerve of the most powerful witch doctor! Jacob had his next operation under general anaesthetic, and turned up smiling for his follow-up visit. Sadly, he dropped out of sight and I was not able to follow his progress as planned.

THE SURGICAL PROCEDURE

Some years ago it was the practice to release tongue tie in very young infants (in the first 6 weeks of life) with thumb pressure on a gauze swab. This would cause momentary distress for the child and a little bleeding which would always rapidly settle.

This method is still sometimes used and is described in detail by Gregory Notestine in his article on the identification of ankyloglossia as a cause of breastfeeding problems.[24]

It is now general practice among the surgeons I have dealt with that surgical release of tongue tie is performed as an elective surgical procedure, in hospital, and under general anaesthesia, when it can be done with great safety, virtually no morbidity, and very little inconvenience to patient and family. The earliest age at which surgery is carried out is usually 6 months. However, when difficulties with breastfeeding occur as a result of a tie, surgery may be performed earlier at the surgeon's discretion.

All the patients who are reported in the study were seen by skilled and experienced surgeons who were interested in tongue tie. The surgeons obtained a speech-therapy report and confirmed the need for an operation which was subsequently performed.

The operation is usually performed on a day–stay basis, with the patient needing to be in hospital for around 3 hours. The operation takes 10 to 15 minutes of this time, and the actual period under anaesthesia is only 4 minutes. The surgical procedures used for children seen as part of the study differ from those described in the available literature, and a description of three techniques used is given in Appendix C.

Operation for tongue tie, although simple by comparison with many other procedures, is never anything but significant and anxiety–provoking to parents and patients. Therefore, recommending surgery must be done with the understanding that it will be a disappointing verdict to those parents who have been hoping that the child merely needs to try harder with his speech. The 'bad news' must be given in an appropriate way. At this juncture, parents need:

- A definite message as to what is recommended. Evasions are misleading and difficult to correct later on.
- Full information and answers to their questions. When available, photographs of the mouths of actual patients, before and after surgery, as well as diagrams, are effective in helping them to grasp the relevant features of the procedure.
- Discussions to address any fears including those of blood transfusions, the risk of HIV, or any other concerns that may be raised.

When it is performed under a general anaesthetic, the whole process can be well controlled, and in spite of the excellent blood supply in the mouth the risk of uncontrollable bleeding is rare, even when the surgeon is not using diathermy.

One of the children in the study was a 'bleeder' who sailed through surgery with no problems. Parents who are worried about the risk of HIV or AIDS may be relieved by donating some of their own blood to be kept for their child should it be required. However, with the techniques described in Appendix C, such a need is highly unlikely.

Parents are obvious candidates for information, but children must not be neglected as they too need to be relaxed about the operation. Many children have fantasies (often based on television) about surgery, the surgeon, anaesthesia and the sleep-inducing injection. Most children see the surgeon as all powerful, even punitive. Children who are grappling with the nature of death may imagine that death is a reversible process, and that they will 'die for a while' during surgery.

It is important to stress that overnight stays are the longest periods for which patients are hospitalised. Most hospitals now have day–stay programmes into which would fall tongue-tie surgery. Fasting before operation is often the most troublesome aspect of the whole experience, particularly for younger children.

RECOVERY AFTER SURGERY
Parents are able to see their children soon after surgery in the Recovery Ward. Some sensitivity of the tongue is common after surgery, and may be worse in older children. All patients can drink soon after the operation and can eat their dinner on the same day. A wide choice of food is open to them. I suggest that hot or spicy foods, such as acid drinks or hot curried dishes be postponed, and that dry toast and crisps are introduced only after the tongue is less sensitive.

Some adults in the study reported muscle pain and felt numbness for up to 10 days. The frenum is much thicker in older subjects and this may be significant. One adult and two children, aged 10 and 12, complained of pain for much longer than others. Two infants with very tight ties, resulting in their tongues being almost fused to the buccal floor, required analgesia for pain on the first day and dribbled profusely. However, in a group of 175 patients who had surgery for tongue tie, pain was not reported to be a problem in the majority of cases.

Healing within the mouth proceeds extremely rapidly and complications are virtually unheard of. The textbooks talk about post-operative haemorrhage but using the techniques described in Appendix C, this has not happened to any of the patients in the study. Patients or parents are warned that the undersurface of the tongue will have a white appearance for a week or so. The absorbable catgut sutures do not require removal. Only the occasional patient is asked to return for routine surgical review. Not all patients have involvement pre-operatively with speech pathologists, but for those that do the family should be urged by the surgeon to arrange speech pathology review post-operatively, and therapy where indicated. Ideally, all patients having surgery for tongue tie should also be assessed by a speech pathologist.

Children in this study have not suffered scar tissue, floppiness of the tongue or excessive pain or bleeding. A second operation was required in only a few cases. One such instance was that of a child with abnormal facial structure, where further loosening was needed after growth had taken place. In this case, a slightly more complex incision—called a Z-plasty—was used the second time. The other cases were those of patients whose ties required repair in stages because of excessive tissue across the floor of the mouth.

DISCOMFORT AFTER SURGERY
Fortunately, unlike major oral surgery such as for cleft lip or palate, the discomfort associated with tongue-tie surgery is fleeting. There are no subsequent painful procedures, no drips or needles, and the advantages quickly become evident. Where stitches are needed because the tie has been very short or tight, the discomfort ensuing may cause dribbling or sensitivity for 2 to 3 days. Absorbable catgut sutures were always used on the children operated on in this study. The following post-operative advice was offered by Whitman and Rankow in 1961 and is still valid today:

> Postoperative care is generally minimal, but the patient may require simple analgesics for pain. Clear fluids may be permitted following complete recovery from the general anaesthetic. No limitations are given regarding motion of the tongue. In fact, tongue motion is encouraged, so as to limit apposition of the transected muscles. If the patient keeps the tongue moving, it is amazing how little soreness or postoperative discomfort he experiences. About one week later, tongue training … should be instituted, since the genioglossotomy, in itself, will not cause the tongue to function properly. The patient must be retrained; otherwise, he will follow the original pattern of malfunction.[26]

Older subjects will sometimes feel more discomfort than toddlers. Excessive salivation and numbness are sometimes temporary symptoms postoperatively. However, patients and parents will quickly forget their earlier fears while appreciating new skills such as licking rather than biting ice creams, chewing a steak or simply being able to eat faster and less messily.

AIMING FOR OPTIMAL SURGERY
The choice of surgical technique is of course the prerogative of the surgeon. It is important that this is not an arbitrary or random choice. It has been my experience that an incision that is too slight makes very little change in the cluster of symptoms, leaving the tongue improved only in appearance, and making prolonged treatment necessary to correct deficits.

In the early post-operative stages, such minimal incisions may seem to have been entirely successful, since freer tongue movement is possible and better feeding or eating patterns are seen. However, over time it becomes evident that diadochokinesis, cosmetic appearance and speech are not significantly changed. The dilemma of when to recommend a second operation (which will undoubtedly be more traumatic for parents and patient) arises. The alternative is to settle for prolonged, and sometimes ineffective, therapy.

Families naturally are disenchanted when they find that a long period of therapy is still required and the speech pathologist may lose some credibility. When speech pathologists recommend surgery, it should be understood that they will also recommend specialist surgeons who are interested in the topic of tongue tie. General practitioners, even those who are surgically experienced, should not be called upon to operate on these patients.

POST-OPERATIVE FINDINGS

In 2 or 3 days, progress in feeding or eating habits becomes apparent: patients eat faster, they accept a wider range of foods, and chewing and swallowing habits improve. Rashes from salivary dribble disappear spontaneously within a week. The need to wash food down with frequent mouthfuls of liquid should also decrease. Weight gain is sometimes quite marked. However, as stressed previously, if feeding has become associated with behavioural problems, progress in this area is slower and counselling may be required.

It was often the case that some insight into a patient's fears and preconceptions was of assistance in enhancing progress. One patient was talking clearly and experimenting with his improved oral function immediately after surgery, until his concerned parent warned him that he had stitches 'in there'. Whereupon he felt very uncomfortable and cut down on all verbal activity for a week!

Some patients with poor oral kinaesthesia become even less competent with exercises and difficult sounds after surgery, when altered mobility of the tongue may give them the illusion of altered oral landmarks. This condition is only temporary, and quickly stabilises when numbness and hypersalivation reduce and specific exercises are practised. However, it can give the impression that the patient's capabilities have deteriorated. Early post-operative follow-ups are essential if such situations (which cannot always be predicted before surgery) are to be managed appropriately.

It was found that children under 5 years could make huge gains immediately after surgery, partic-

ularly if they had been receiving speech therapy—however non-productive it may have appeared—before the operation. As soon as lingual mobility was provided, oral kinaesthesia improved very rapidly and homework tasks now produced a sense of achievement, rather than failure.

Marcus was 18 months when he had surgery for obvious tongue tie and poverty of language (he communicated in grunts). His mother reported that in the first week after surgery he used five or six new words and he appeared to be much happier. From the second week on, his vocabulary grew larger every day. He began regularly using two words together, and often used three. He talked constantly and used all aspects of language: nouns, adjectives, adverbs and verbs.

Older children frequently complain of pain after surgery. While this may be explained by thickening of the tie in older subjects, greater complication of the surgery, or mature understanding leading to heightened apprehension, there is also the fact that the older child has been handicapped by his weak organ for longer, and has developed certain behaviours around it. He is used to his symptoms and sometimes derives secondary gains from them.

A sudden change in the 'status quo' can also cause anxiety in overprotected children, who are then acutely conscious of every post-operative twinge.

In summary, surgical intervention has many advantages: the simplicity of the procedure, a short hospital stay, quick recovery time and consistency in terms of results. Obviously the expertise of the surgeon is important, but this applies to all such procedures, whether simple or complicated. When combined with appropriate speech therapy, the improvement in speech and oromuscular function seen post-operatively in patients in the study speaks volumes for the potential of surgical release as a treatment for tongue tie.

6   Speech Therapy after Surgery

The importance of post-operative follow-up by a speech pathologist cannot be over-stressed. Some surgeons order it routinely, others only request it for those patients who have particularly difficult problems. Periodic speech pathology follow-up should routinely be arranged, unless the patient is already engaged in ongoing therapy, when post-operative follow-up and re-assessment can be part of the therapeutic process.

It is recommended that the assessment method described in Appendix B is used at post-operative review of all patients at 2 weeks, 3 months and 6 months after surgery. This makes it possible to monitor progress, to reduce anxiety, and to deal with any problems that occur along the way before they become entrenched. If normal speech has not been acquired during this time, or if problems with dribbling or feeding are persisting or are causing anxiety, speech therapy should be commenced. Many children under 3 years will need no more than post-operative follow-up appointments, but older children and adults will probably need ongoing therapy.

Some parents are unrealistic in their expectations due to lack of information, and will, if unchecked, give unnecessarily negative or impossibly optimistic guidelines to their children. Regular follow-ups are a vital part of good management of tongue tie. However, it must be stressed to parents that surgery alone will not correct all the problems associated with the condition, which occur in patients who are past infancy at the time of intervention.

It was found repeatedly that as a consequence of disordered oromuscular functioning, poor oral kinaesthesia and limited lingual mobility, the patient over the age of 3 years was unable to correct faulty patterns of movement unaided. These would persist after successful division of the frenum unless suitable therapy was undertaken.

No model for post-operative speech therapy for patients with tongue tie has previously been devised because surgery was generally seen as failing to help these patients and has been less regarded as a therapeutic measure. However, my study has shown conclusively that with surgery and suitable techniques of therapy, patients can and do acquire normal speech and functions.

Some authorities in the field of dentistry promoted a combination of surgery and therapy years ago. It is interesting that Ketty and Sciullo recommend that: 'Surgery, if indicated, should be performed in the preschool years to allow the child to undergo tongue exercises and speech therapy.'[3]

Describing an operation for tongue tie in a 24-year-old patient, Douglas and Kresberg say:

> The surgical procedure in this case was important, but without adequate guidance this patient may never have had any improvement in function. Speech impediments do not 'correct themselves' and the training with a speech therapist post-operatively helped to acquire the desired result.[30]

When speech therapy was required, it was found that the main thrust of therapy needed to be in the area of oral kinaesthesia. Experience has shown that the severe consequences of limited tongue movement on the development of oral kinaesthesia affect oromuscular function and prevent the acquisition of correct swallowing patterns. This results in very poor diadochokinesis in all patients with tongue tie. Happily, this can be effectively overcome with the management described in Chapter 6.

Fletcher and Meldrum, writing about a comparison of articulatory proficiency in two groups of children with and without tongue tie, said:

> Significant differences were found between these two groups both in speech articulation errors and in diadochokinetic rates of movement ... These findings are particularly pertinent to the clinical entity called congenital inferior ankyloglossia or Tongue tie.[10]

Williams and Waldron sum it up nicely:

> It seems reasonable to hypothesise that physical restriction of the tongue might limit the speed with which the tongue can be moved.[8]

It is the case that diverse opinions are available in the literature and in practice, and that these are based largely on individual experience and theory. However, when all available data are assembled, it becomes impossible to doubt either the reality of the problems associated with this condition, or the efficacy of relevant surgery when it is accompanied by speech therapy.

THE CRITICAL AGE
It has been stated already that many children who have surgery under the age of 3 years are able to acquire normal speech, improve feeding habits, and gradually adopt normal oromuscular movement without the need for regular speech therapy. Subsequently, tongue posture and shape also become normal. The typical blunt-ended tongue gradually becomes pointed, and oral kinaesthetic skills improve spontaneously with time.

Children under the age of three generally acquired the pointed tongue tip and improved oromuscular function spontaneously after surgery, together with improved speech. They were followed up at intervals of 1, 3 and 6 months. Where there were no behaviour problems, feeding habits improved in 1 week, and mothers reported faster eating, acceptance of a wider range of textures and an ability to suck from straws after the operation. Sadly, children whose tongue tie was diagnosed later, or whose operations had been postponed, took much longer to overcome feeding idiosyncrasies. As with so many developmental skills, behavioural aspects had come into play and secondary gains and habits combined to keep them well entrenched.

LATE OPERATION
Patients who have surgery after the age of three need speech therapy for the most serious consequence of their tongue tie: an underdeveloped oral kinaesthetic sense. This is the problem which underlies all the symptoms observers note when they see and hear a patient with tongue tie. It leads to a lack of awareness of the geography of the mouth; results in poverty of lingual, sensory and locomotor experiences; contributes to feeding and speech problems; and produces oral movements which are poorly controlled and limited in range and variety (see Plate 21). In general, the older the patient at the time of operation, the more significant the kinaesthetic deficit.

Surprisingly few articles referring to this aspect of tongue tie were found in the literature. Although there were references to articulatory problems which were hypothetically attributed to many causes—ranging from agenesis of the tongue tip, congenital supra bulbar palsy, dyspraxia, and hypoplasia of the tongue tip, to 'other causes'—kinaesthesia was mentioned in only two articles as a cause of articulatory difficulty.

Fletcher and Meldrum, and Williams and Waldron, all assessed lingual function in patients with ankyloglossia using tests of diadochokinesis and measurements of the size and configuration of the tongue and frenum. Williams and Waldron comment that 'a generalised disorder of oral motor function will likely appear in labial as well as lingual function.'[8]

AFTER SURGERY
It is suggested that exercises are commenced 1 week after operation, and are graded according to discomfort, i.e. 'stop when it hurts or when you get tired'. Ten minutes of practice twice daily is more effective than half-an-hour at irregular intervals.

Although I have recommended that therapy starts 1 week after surgery, some patients are unwilling to wait. One 10-year-old was so determined to get rid of all his embarrassing lingual deficiencies that he practised the exercises from the day after surgery, whenever he could. When seen 5 days after surgery he had made progress that other patients took months to achieve! He had increased his range of tongue movements, and when reviewed in 1 month he had acquired a point on his tongue—a stage that is usually arrived at only after 3 months of regular practice. In this case no unwanted consequences ensued but, in general, it is probably wiser to postpone commencement of exercises.

Gentle exercise after the operation is vital for all patients. As Whitman and Rankow advise: 'tongue movement is encouraged, so as to limit apposition of the transected muscles.'[26]

However, with the modern techniques described in Appendix C, knitting together of raw edges is unlikely to occur. Rogers and Douglas made these comments about post-operative progress:

The sutures were removed 2 days after operation and the patient was instructed to exercise his tongue freely, particularly in extension and prefer-ably in front of a mirror. One week following the operation, he was able to touch the lingual surfaces of the upper teeth and the rugae palatinae.[32]

As mentioned earlier, absorbable catgut sutures are now used, so that stitches no longer need to be removed after operation.

POST–OPERATIVE FOLLOW–UP
Speech therapy after surgery should be related to results on the assessment tasks. This sets concrete goals for patients. It allows the speech pathologist to home in on areas of weakness identified pre-operatively, and to monitor the results of surgery and therapy.

Task specific oromuscular exercises should be commenced immediately after assessment, and are of benefit when practised regularly even before surgery. Post-operatively, exercises should be continued on a daily basis until function is satisfactory.

Parents should be urged to get into the routine of monitoring and encouraging homework exercises as soon as the diagnosis has been made. Practice routines should be established while motivation is high and before the impact of diagnosis and assessment can wear off. Familiarity with the exercises also gives parents more understanding of the peculiar difficulties of tongue tie—helping them to be tolerant rather than critical of their child's failures.

Using a mirror, the patient can begin building up oral-kinaesthetic sense even before surgery has provided greater freedom of lingual movement. Repetition of the simple task specific exercises devised, with visual and auditory monitoring of the resulting sounds produced, has been found to assist in building up oral kinaesthesia, and teaching patients how to plan and attempt desired oral and lingual movements.

Even small children will benefit from these exercises before surgery. I have often been told by interested parents that a child is progressing with a particular skill before the operation. The progress made is not such as to induce patients to refuse surgery and a well prepared patient or parent is not likely to change his mind in the interim. On the contrary, success spurs them on to anticipate greater lingual freedom. Having become familiar with the exercises before operation, patients are less tentative when performing them after surgery.

ORAL HYGIENE

More frequent swallowing habits have to be specifically taught, since poor oral kinaesthesia will have prevented the patient from realising when it is time to dispose of excess saliva by swallowing. At the post-operative interview, gums and teeth should be checked, and questions asked about oral hygiene. Specific exercises should be included for clearing food off the surfaces of the teeth, with tongue movements.

FEEDING

Often, because of difficulties with mastication and manipulation of food, the patient has persisted with a limited range of foods, food fads, infantilised feeding, prolonged breastfeeding or pureeing of foods.

One 18-month-old child seen was still on the breast, because she had been unable to tolerate even ground foods until she was 10 months old. One mouthful of pureed food would cause her to gag repeatedly, a violent reaction which forced her parents to rely on breastfeeding as her main source of nourishment .

Another little boy was breastfed until he was 2 years and 6 months old because he could not be nourished in any other way—he gagged and choked on all other forms of food. Changing this emphasis post-operatively would naturally be unpopular with the patient and worrying to the

mother who would need to be supported through any attempts she made to normalise feeding. Change would need to occur quite gradually.

Feeding and eating can be monitored from discussions with the parent or adult patient and particular problems addressed. A great deal of attention will need to be directed towards tongue-thrust swallowing. A myofunctional-tongue therapy programme may be used, but the speech pathologist will need to be selective about which exercises are recommended. Very detailed and demanding exercises, which cannot be mastered in the early post-operative period, predictably cause frustration and loss of co-operation.

It is imperative that anomalies in feeding be addressed, because the development of good chewing, sucking and swallowing will form the basis of desirable speech patterns. Parents must be advised and supported through the exigencies of increasing the intake of solids, reducing liquid intake to age-appropriate levels and promoting socially acceptable chewing and swallowing. Several children seen for the purposes of the study had been breastfed for inordinate lengths of time because they were unable to change existing patterns of sucking and swallowing, and thus could not drink from a cup or be adequately nourished with solid supplements. Mothers were consequently being labelled as infantilising the child or even being self-indulgent.

The infantile or tongue-thrust swallow must be assessed, and when present in children old enough to carry out specific tongue exercises, swallowing with the tongue pressing on the hard palate must be practised. Younger children can benefit from an indirect attack on the problem: play involving tongue pointing, clicks, and the Mr Tongue Story *(see Appendix D)* may be used to facilitate a pointed, upward-oriented tongue in action.

As noted earlier, Teurk and Lubit believe that inability to raise the tongue to the roof of the palate may prevent development of an adult swallow and lead to an open bite, malocclusion, and hence mandibular prognathism.[3] However, these opinions are not accepted by all and undoubtedly more research is needed to clarify the position.

LINGUAL MOVEMENTS

My clinical observations have demonstrated that elevation of the tongue to the upper lip, or the alveolar ridge, is the hardest skill to master. Although contact can be made with the lips almost shut, opening the jaws appears to cause the patient to lose the sense of space and direction, and the tongue flops. The tongue tends to remain blunt-ended, until enough strong, pointing movements have been made to register the 'pointed shape memory' on the brain. In most patients this took 3 months with regular daily practice. The slight notching on the tongue margin remains as a permanent feature, yet causes no problems. For a comparison of attempts at elevation before and after surgery, see Plates 23 and 24, respectively.

ORAL KINAESTHESIA

Large diagrams may be used to instruct the patient in the geography of the mouth and in how particular sounds are made. A brief categorisation of sounds is often useful: vowels, consonants, plosives, nasals, sibilants, etc. The patient is asked to visualise the oral space, and to touch or trace drawings representing the lips, tongue or palate at their points of articulation for different sounds and in targeted words, while saying the words at varying speeds and volumes.

SPEECH

Speech therapy must be very flexible, yet the speech exercises set must be task specific. This requires some experience in judging the nature and severity of the child's problem and the ability to select, from a range of tasks, the one that is likely to

be mastered and hence be non-threatening. Patients with tongue tie have already experienced failure in many basic areas of their lives, while remaining outside the range of sympathy by having an unrecognised handicap. Speech pathologists should avoid adding to their experiences of failure.

I vividly remember being asked to give a second opinion on a boy with mild cerebral palsy and a very severe tongue tie, who dribbled continuously while he tried valiantly to push a large wooden block over the desk with his tongue. This exercise had been recommended to strengthen tongue control, but I felt it was much more likely to cause him to rip the frenum with his sharp little milk teeth. He could not stretch his tongue any further because of the tie, and could only use the blade of the tongue for pushing, but was being asked to achieve the impossible for theoretical, rather than realistic, reasons.

It is essential that speech-therapy tasks provide some concrete experience of success. The exercises used should be simple, staggered for difficulty, and fun to do. The speech pathologist should begin and end the exercise with easy tasks, and develop variations on the earlier tasks that provide more kinaesthetic challenges.

Mirrors, line drawings, and colour photographs assist in visualisation of the oral space. Pacing spoken words with a metronome, and finger tapping or clapping help in speeding up speech that is correct at slow rates but quite disconnected at speed; tape recordings can be used to facilitate changes from loud to soft voice, or to elaborate isolated sounds, and to assist the patient to make chains of repeated sounds.

Specific sound errors must also be dealt with, using conventional speech therapy methods.

It is often necessary to teach the patient to open his or her mouth sufficiently when speaking. Patients who cannot make articulatory contacts during connected speech, because they have difficulty reaching a specific oral target in a hurry, often defend against error by speaking through half-closed teeth; they are still unclear, but know instinctively that they cannot reach the required point of articulatory contact, and so will continue to resist opening their mouths in case they lose all their 'landmarks'.

Often children with tongue tie have a history of having started talking with acceptably clear single words. Subsequently, they make small sentences, but as the demands of their growing language require them to talk faster, think more, use longer sentences and harder words, they become unable to co-ordinate all these operations. Any added stress—be it louder or faster speech, or emotion—makes it impossible for them to speak clearly.

Whitman and Rankow describe the tongue training that they do with their patients. They say the hard palate is pressed with a blunt instrument, about in line with the first permanent molars. Then a small irregular piece of sugarless mint is placed in the hollow formed in the anterior third of the tongue. The patient is asked to close his or her teeth and hold the candy on the spot on the roof of the mouth which was previously touched. When he or she finds the proper position the 'tongue will no longer protrude between or press against, the teeth. … This exercise is to be done constantly for the next 3 or 4 days. The reason for doing it constantly is that one swallows during all of his waking hours. A little training now and then will do absolutely no good.'[26]

Reducing concomitant movements of the head when performing lingual tasks (see Plate 19) has to be taught using a mirror, as has maintaining the tongue at rest when not speaking.

Tongue elevation can sometimes be taught by asking the child to touch the alveolar ridge with the lips shut, then sliding the tongue out of the mouth, and then carefully parting the lips. However, until the patient is able to isolate tongue-elevating and mouth-opening movements, this task can not be considered to have been accomplished.

THERAPEUTIC PROGNOSIS

Children with tongue tie show patchy progress; long periods of fruitless struggle are punctuated with sudden successes, when it seems 'the penny drops' and a particular task is mastered. Once this has happened, the task or movement is rarely lost. Unlike teaching a sibilant 's' for instance, which may be forgotten over a break in therapy, acquiring this new skill seems to indicate a kinaesthetic milestone, which is then internalised permanently. However, this generalisation applies more to movements than to speech sounds, which seem to be more complex, incorporating both auditory and tactile feedback.

When correcting speech sounds, which involve auditory skills, it takes longer to introduce these into normal use than to acquire a new movement. Once these successes begin to occur there is a gradual acceleration of the rate of progress, as oral kinaesthesia gets better and better and the child begins to tap into these skills spontaneously to achieve his goals.

However, if there are associated problems such as developmental delay, hearing loss, or severe emotional disturbance, this spontaneous recovery takes longer to occur, or does not occur at all, and longer speech therapy is required. Patients with conditions such as cerebral palsy or hearing loss will have different patterns of recovery, depending on the particular features of their disability.

One child with cerebral palsy, who had surgery, initially showed very little change in the speech area. Then she gradually began to close her lips for swallowing. Previously she had been unable to retrieve food, which would get stuck on the palate and later become loosened, falling off the palate and causing gagging and vomiting. This ceased

2 weeks after operation and enlargement of vocabulary occurred slowly thereafter. Improved emotional stability and reduction of catastrophic reactions occurred in 4 weeks and the patient now communicates verbally although with pronunciation difficulties.

WHEN INTENSIVE THERAPY IS REQUIRED

The older the patient at time of operation, the more significant the kinaesthetic deficit. Unfortunately, there is often an expectation on the part of the older child that surgery will provide a miracle cure. The resultant disappointment can often complicate future therapy and needs tactful handling.

I have found the shape of the tongue in patients with tongue tie to be indicative of the movements of which it is capable. A thick, blunt-ended, slow-moving tongue will produce neither precise movements, nor the huge variations of shape, that normal tongues must produce in speech. Often patients with moderately severe ties and poor speech would present with an unusually broad, flat tongue with a long point in the middle. The presence of the point could lead to the tongue tie being judged to be 'mild'. The tongue in these instances tends to be overactive and unable to hold a posture, and the point disappears in speech, so that lingual contacts continue to be thickened and lispy *(see Plate 4)*.

It was found that encouraging the child to aim at producing a pointed tongue, and having the patient practice exercises that require tongue pointing, aiming, and graded and controlled movement, assisted in developing oral kinaesthesia and did more than anything else to promote good oromuscular function after surgery.

It is a very striking fact that all children with tongue tie who were of normal intelligence were able to identify the tasks they were unable to perform, even on their first visit. They would count aloud slowly but refuse to attempt faster rates.

Toddlers, happily employed in a game of making faces, would imitate all movements, but sulk and cling to their mother if asked to protrude their tongues horizontally. They were well aware that they could protrude their tongues downwards but not horizontally, and that they could not elevate the tongue to the alveolar ridge. Obviously they were also aware of confusion in regard to orientation in the oral space and needed to learn this. Thus, providing lingual mobility without following it up with therapy would be inadequate intervention.

Speech therapy for tongue tie is particularly challenging, because here we find a blend of factors, each of which could cause a speech problem on its own. There may be genetic factors, organic weakness or limitation, factors of habit, faulty speech patterns based on foundations of poor feeding in infancy, and emotional reactions to the frustrations and limitations of tongue tie. In each case the strength or weakness of the different elements vary, depending on age or other circumstances. Each patient's case must be treated individually. Speech symptoms may relate to one or more factors, such as articulation, voice, fluency or development of language. Sometimes there are also other problems, such as associated hearing loss or developmental delay.

When surgery has been successfully performed the potential for a really successful outcome is excellent, and thus the effort is in most cases very rewarding for patients, their families, the speech pathologists and the surgeons. Neither surgery nor speech therapy alone is likely to prove an adequate or successful form of intervention, with the possible exception of early surgical release in the case of an infant who has no other disabilities, congenital or acquired, which are equally likely to cause speech difficulty. In the course of my study it became clear that a combination of surgery and speech therapy is required for the effective treatment of most cases of tongue tie.

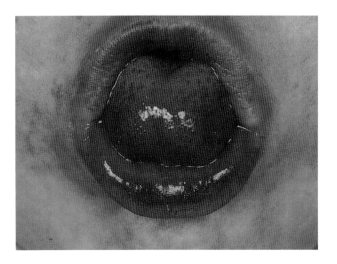

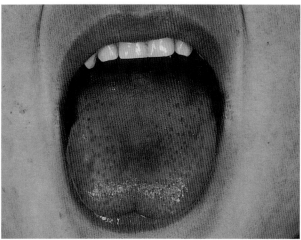

Plate 1

The tongue looks conspicuously 'different'. Note the rectangular block of lingual tissue, and the rash a round the lips from salivary debris.

Plate 2

Notching of the lingual margin produces a typical heart-shaped tongue. Dimpling marks the point of insertion of the restraining genioglossus muscle.

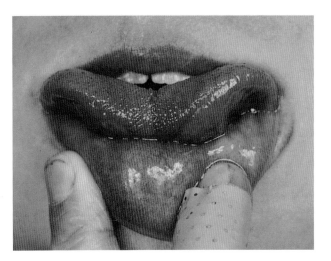

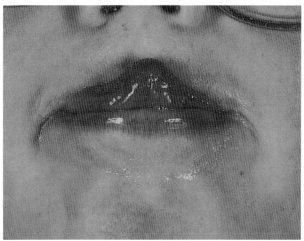

Plate 3

There is no tongue tip, and the bulging upward-curving sides of the tongue and overflowing saliva, are visible in extra-oral elevation.

Plate 4

The tongue has a small tip, in this 'mild tie' which permits elevation, but it must be gripped by the lips, during movement. Note saliva.

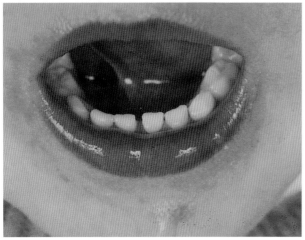

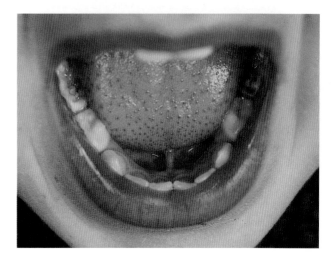

Plate 5
A thin transparent membranous tie prevents necessary swallowing of saliva, and causes a salivary rash in a 5-year-old.

Plate 6
A short, thick tie shown by retraction of the tongue. Dental caries and pooled saliva visible.

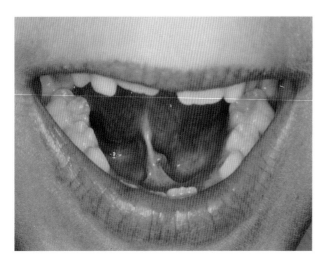

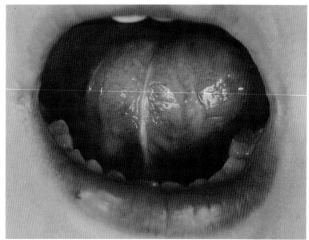

Plate 7
Extending to the lower front teeth this short tie shows a lingual frenal epithelioma caused by trauma from the lower incisors.

Plate 8
A thick tie deeply embedded in lingual tissue. The tongue is broad, flat and leaf-like with active sides.

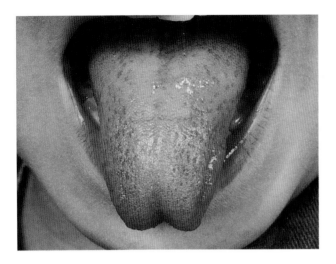

Plate 9

The tongue 'tip' is pulled down on strong downward protrusion, which is possible even with some severe ties. Indentation of the lingual margin results.

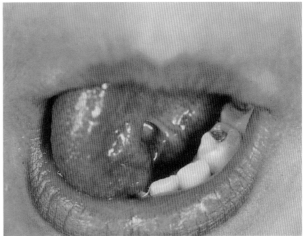

Plate 10

This tongue cannot stretch far in any direction. A very short tie causes tongue rolling during movement. Dental caries and hypersalivation are obvious.

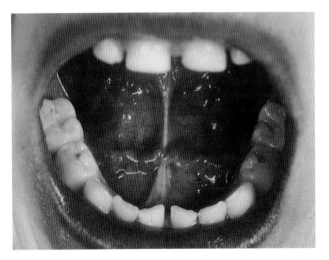

Plate 11

A fan-shaped tie extends to the lower incisors, but permits limited elevation. Dental plaque and excess saliva are visible.

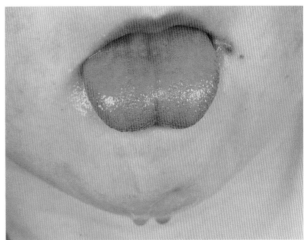

Plate 12

Poor oral hygiene causes a rash around the mouth due to spilling of saliva. This was the only voluntary movement that could be made by the patient.

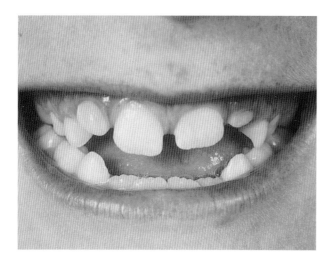

Plate 13
Irregular dentition, and an open bite, with the tongue resting on the lower front teeth at rest, and when swallowing.

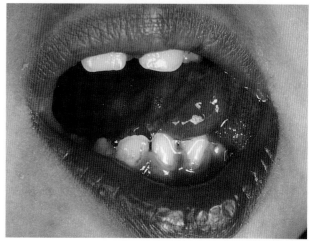

Plate 14
Bizarre movements made during attempts at lateral licking, show the tongue curling while the lip and jaw push sideways with effort.

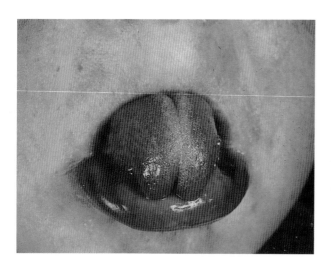

Plate 15
An effort at protrusion causes a central lingual fissure and hypersalivation. The lips are needed to help to immobilise the tongue, as the strongest pull on the tie occurs in this movement.

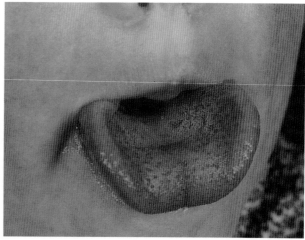

Plate 16
The middle of the tongue is anchored, the sides are active and wide, and muscles around the mouth contract to keep the tongue still.

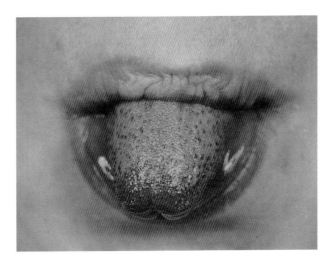

Plate 17
An uncertain attempt at downward pointing. The tongue extends for a considerable distance with effort in this posture, despite the tie.

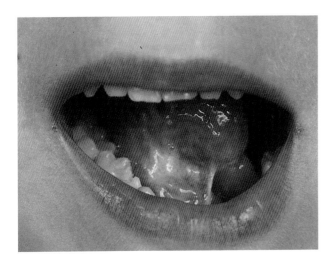

Plate 18
The tongue tie is too tight to allow the tongue to reach the inside corner of the mouth, though the jaw pushes sideways to help.

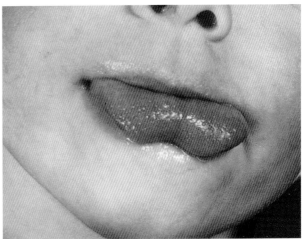

Plate 19
The head tilts sideways to help in lateral pointing outside the mouth, but the tip is pulled under and cannot reach the corner.

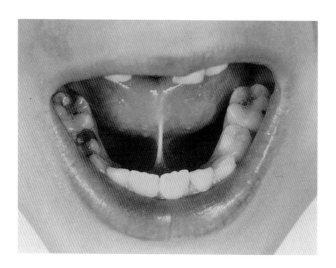

Plate 20
Retraction of the tongue allows a short thick fan-shaped tie, to be seen.

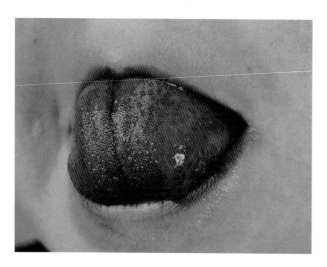

Plate 21
Without visual clues, a sluggish, under-active tongue can only make non-specific, perseverative movements during assessment.

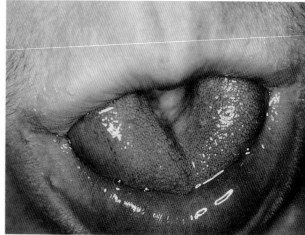

Plate 22
A teenager with unsightly tongue and uncontrolled salivation suffers both physically and emotionally.

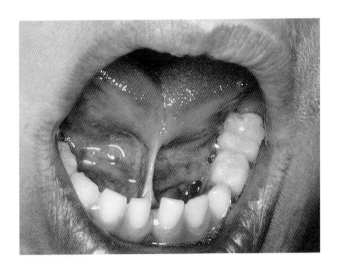

Plate 23
Attempt at elevation of the tongue, before surgery.

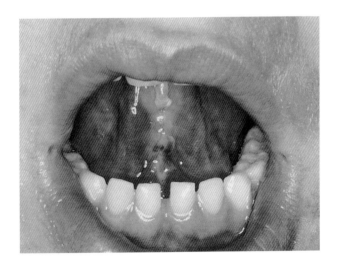

Plate 24
Attempt at elevation of the tongue, after surgery.

Illustrations to be used with 'Mr. Tongue' Story
(page 76)

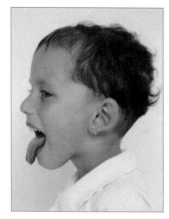

Plate 25
He stretched

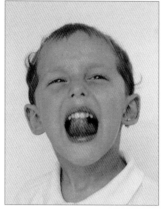

Plate 26
He reached up

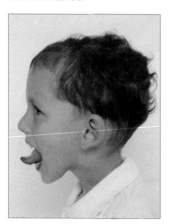

Plate 27
He went past the fence

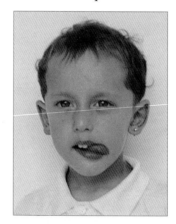

Plate 28
He looked to the left

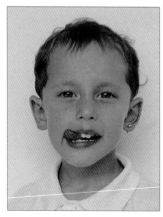

Plate 29
He looked to the right

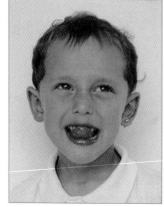

Plate 30
Up the road

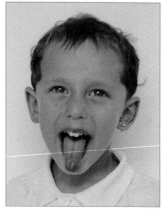

Plate 31
He went down the road

7   Case Histories

INTRODUCTION

The case histories presented in this chapter were selected from the 200 cases that were assessed during the study. They are all clear examples of some of the significant and important aspects of tongue-tie management.

Each history illustrates a particular facet of the tongue-tie picture and has led to the development of a hypothesis regarding appropriate management of the condition. The hypothesis is further elucidated by background information, assessment data, and a column chart illustrating the improvement achieved following surgery and speech therapy.

Figure 1 represents a composite picture of the 10 case histories described in this chapter and compares the total TAP scores, before and after intervention, for each of the patients.

Figure 1

Comparison of total TAP scores before and after intervention

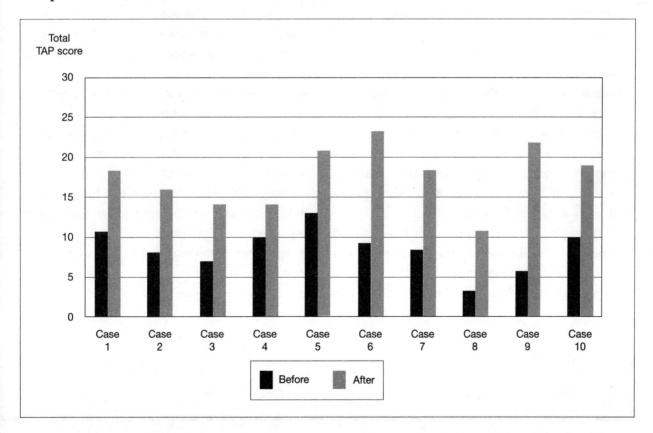

Case History 1:

Optimal Management of Tongue Tie

Hypothesis

Most children under the age of three who have surgery for tongue tie develop speech normally. They need regular reviews to monitor progress and to ensure that all areas of communication are developing well but prolonged speech therapy is not required.

History

Jon was first seen when aged 18 months. His tongue tie was noted at birth. He was breastfed for 4 days only, and bottle fed for 10 months. His mother did not feel that he had a feeding problem at any stage.

Observations

Cosmetic appearance: The tie was easily seen as it extended to the anterior lingual margin and had been observed at birth.

Oral hygiene and dental health: No unusual amount of dribbling noted, but as there was limited lingual activity and firm lip closure, excess of saliva may well have been hidden.

Feeding skills: He was reported to have a good appetite, he could chew chicken and meat, but could not lick an ice cream.

Lingual movement: Very little lingual activity was seen during assessment. The patient attempted to comply with requests for tongue movement, by using fingers to aid in tongue protrusion, and failed. Horizontal protrusion was possible up to the mucobuccal fold only. No elevation of the tongue was possible but he would attempt to assist it by lifting his chin. Lingual protrusion downwards was attempted and failed. No lateral movements were seen. Full circumlocution was not seen as the tongue was incapable of elevation, and only the lower lip could be touched.

Oral kinaesthesia: This aspect could not be tested, because of the patient's age, but he appeared to be aware of the movements that he was unable to copy.

Speech: He was reported to know and use 23 single words at home, but the only words heard during assessment were 'no mummy, no' angrily, when he failed to stick out his tongue as requested.

Emotional status: Jon presented as a happy, docile child till speech or tongue movements were requested. He was clearly confident in all areas except those involving oral or lingual function. He expressed frustration and refused to try the lingual movements he knew he could not do.

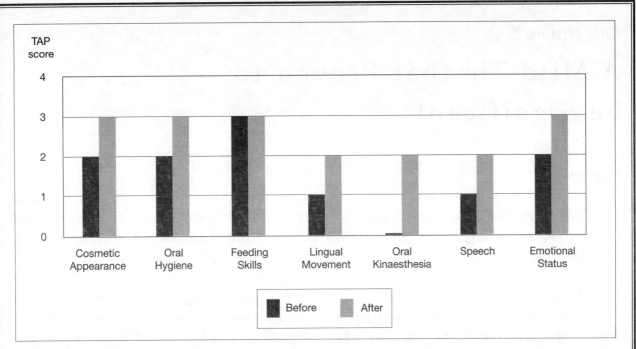

Figure 2

Comparison of total TAP scores before and after intervention

Progress

The pre-operative total TAP score was 11.

Exercises to increase the scope of oral play were prescribed pre-operatively, and surgery was recommended.

When seen 1 month after surgery the patient had acquired many new words and was already attempting to use phrases. He was singing, and experimenting spontaneously with tongue play and clicks. He now chewed with lips closed, and dribbling (although not obviously excessive before operation) was noted to have reduced, until he started teething again. He was willing to demonstrate lingual movements and was described as more mature.

His earliest post-operative total TAP score was 18.

Conclusions

This patient did not need regular therapy as he progressed steadily with only periodic reviews for the purpose of monitoring his recovery. Early diagnosis and intervention before the critical age of 3 years resulted in the spontaneous acquisition of normal communicative skills. When followed up again at age four he was achieving well in all areas, and talking fluently and clearly. He then achieved a total TAP score of 21.

Case History 2:

A Mild Tie that Proved to be Significant

Hypothesis

A patient with tongue tie may present with only a mild limitation of tongue movement, but could well be severely handicapped through the cumulative effects of tongue tie.

History

Leif was referred for speech therapy when he was 5 years old. His tongue tie had been observed at birth, but judged to be insignificant. It was eventually diagnosed after 6 months of speech therapy, that was judged to have been unsuccessful.

Observations

Cosmetic appearance: This aspect was not strikingly different, however the tongue was thin, broad and flat during use and the sides of the tongue were unusually active. The tie showed as a thickened white membrane attached at the midpoint of the tongue, but did not impress as tight.

Oral hygiene and dental health: He was prone to dribble and splash saliva. The patient's ability to clean food off his teeth was obviously inadequate. Leif often had food debris around his mouth after a meal, and always looked wet and bubbly about the lips.

Feeding skills: Leif was breastfed for 10 months and then went on to a cup. Now, at 5 years, he drank copiously and frequently, sucked from a straw and, apparently, chewed well.

Lingual movement: The tongue was long and could achieve pointing, but was generally broad and flattened in use. Tongue movements during speech were minimal, but at rest Leif made constant thrusting, uncontrolled lingual movements and sucked his tongue. All movements required during assessment had been learnt during his therapy, and could be performed on demand. However they were not used with any consistency during speech. These learned movements could not be repeated accurately, and tongue positions could not be maintained for more than a few seconds.

Oral kinaesthesia: This was poor, even with visual feedback, (e.g. when watching the speech pathologist or looking in a mirror), and this deficit seriously impeded the progress of therapy. Leif made strong clumsy tongue movements and could not easily alter their direction or control the force of lingual movement.

Speech: Intelligibility was variable. DDK was so poor, that Leif was unable to co-ordinate three consonants in speech exercises, even at slow speeds. It was inevitable that this child's presentation would suggest an emotional rather than an organic aetiology, as there were many observably immature behaviours.

Emotional status: His behaviour was strongly regressive and dependent, although he was a

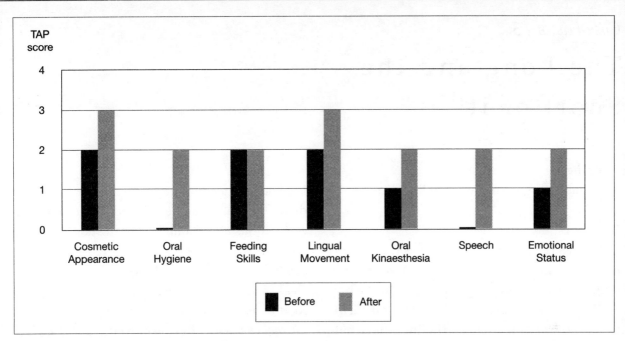

Figure 3

Comparison of total TAP scores before and after intervention

very intelligent child. Delayed success with speech therapy contributed to his unmotivated attitude. He was manipulative, stubborn and generally silent, and resisted passively during all speech therapy experiences. He was still eneuretic at 5 years.

Progress

The pre-operative total TAP score was 8.

Following surgery, there was dramatic progress. Leif became co-operative, interested, and successful within a week. Salivation came under control rapidly, and in 3 months DDK and articulation had improved to the point where regular speech therapy was discontinued at his mother's request. However, in view of the habit formation involved in his previous poor speech patterns, continuation of home practice was strongly recommended.

A post-operative total TAP score of 16 was obtained at discharge.

Conclusion

Lief's 'mild' tongue tie caused a wide range of apparently behaviourial symptoms which did not respond to therapy. The pathological effects in cases of so-called 'mild tongue tie' can be mainly emotional, mainly physiological, or a blend of the two. Frequently, such a cluster of symptoms is attributed to an emotional cause rather than to the consequences of organic aetiology. Removal of the organic factor brought instant improvement by consolidation of the earlier speech therapy efforts.

Case History 3:

The Long and the Short of it!

Hypothesis

Inadequate surgical release is of little benefit.

History

Colin was referred because of speech and feeding problems thought to be caused by his tongue tie. Seen at the age of 18 months he had a history of unregarded early feeding difficulty. He even dribbled when drinking from a bottle. He was subject to upper respiratory tract infections.

The tongue tie was familial, with both paternal and maternal grandmothers and a paternal second cousin being affected. At birth, his tongue was described as looking like a serpent's tongue. Colin was a child of above average intelligence, his parents had easy access to medical information, and the tie had been noted soon after birth. Despite these positive factors, the wide-ranging consequences of the condition had not been realised.

Observations

Cosmetic appearance: Colin had a bulky tongue with the tip curled under by a short thick tie.

Oral hygiene and dental health: This aspect was very poor. Colin had always dribbled a lot, he ate messily, and frequently had a rash around his mouth from salivary residue.

Feeding skills: He was breastfed up until 11 months, and was initially described as not hav

ing had any feeding problems. However, it was discovered later that he still had significant difficulty in this area. Colin had been subject to colic until he was 4 months old. He fed better with solids, but although he chewed tenderised meat, steak and chicken, he often could not contain food in his mouth while chewing.

Lingual movement: Tongue movement was severely limited. Colin was unable to lick, and unable to protrude, elevate or move the tongue laterally. The tongue tended to sit low in the mouth, so that the lower jaw was often protruded beyond the upper. Colin could not kiss his mother; instead, he used to blow.

Oral kinaesthesia: This function was also poor and Colin could not judge direction or grade oral movements.

Speech: At the age of 18 months, Colin had 10 vestigial single words which he used repeatedly and imaginatively, with much gesture so as to increase their meaning. Initial and final consonants both tended to be omitted, so meaning was implied by voice, gestures and context. He had a loud, deep and husky voice which was barely ever inflected, and which also became hoarse with over-use when he was frustrated.

Emotional status: Colin was a charming and affectionate child, but he was also very self willed and easily angered. He disliked and avoided being controlled, and made this very clear at all times.

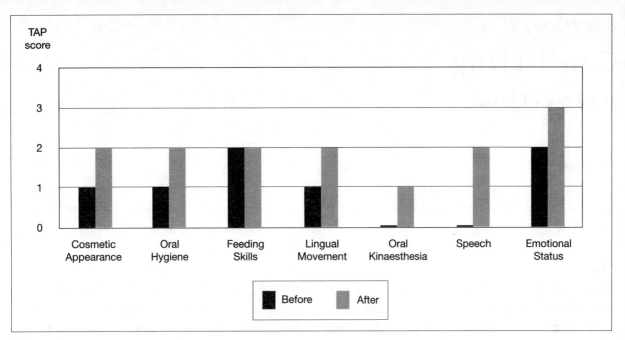

Figure 4
Comparison of total TAP scores before and after intervention

Progress

His pre-operative total TAP score was 7.

Against the speech pathologist's advice, Colin was taken to a surgeon unfamiliar with tongue tie. Following surgery, Colin initially made dramatic progress, exploring the oral space lingually, and using phrases to communicate. His need to drink during meals became less. However, at 2 years and 4 months, although using 5-word phrases and still having speech therapy, his speech remained very unclear, and movement and oral kinaesthesia did not progress further.

His voice was still rough and loud, and showed signs of effortful production. The frenum could still be seen as a thick white cord, which permitted poorly controlled movement but looked conspicuously different. Tongue movements were deliberate and clumsy and an infantile swallow and husky voice persisted for 4 years.

Speech therapy was continued, on and off, until Colin was 7 years old, as his parents preferred this to a second operation. Although still friendly and charming, a hasty impatient temper and overly strong reactions to frustration continued to be part of his personality.

He was finally discharged with a post-operative total TAP score of 14.

Conclusions

Inadequate surgical release of a tongue tie will result in cosmetic improvement and some increase in mobility. However, oral kinaesthesia and speech are unlikely to improve and even after prolonged speech therapy, the patient will continue to function as if he had a moderate tongue tie. Personality is often affected as a result of prolongation of the speech impediment.

Case History 4:

Conflicting Priorities

Hypothesis

When associated problems such as cleft palate take priority, a child may be left very handicapped by a severe tongue tie.

History

Maggie, aged 7 years, had a well-repaired cleft of the hard and soft palates. All early feeding problems had been attributed solely to her cleft palate. She had, predictably, suffered from many upper respiratory tract infections, probably due to aspiration of fluids. However, when seen she fed competently, although slowly.

Observations

Cosmetic appearance: The tongue was flat and broad, with a large notch in the lingual margin and a short, tight, clearly visible tie. Cosmetically, her appearance was very poor with malocclusion and open-mouthed posture.

Oral hygiene and dental health: Limitation of tongue movement contributed to poor oral hygiene. Food debris collected in her mouth, and a ring of food would be seen around her mouth after meals. Maggie had an open bite and breathed through her mouth. She was undergoing orthodontia. There was poor control of saliva during speech.

Feeding skills: Due to the presence of cleft palate all anomalies of feeding were attributed to the major problem. However, Maggie continued to be slow at eating, in spite of good repair of the palate

performed at appropriate stages of development. *Lingual movement:* All tongue movements could be made on request, as a result of earlier speech therapy, but were slow and careful and needed effort. Protrusion of the tongue was limited and difficult. Elevation of the tongue and protrusion downwards could be performed accurately but the movements needed to be deliberate. Lateral movements and circumlocution were found difficult, and to perform these Maggie had to support the tongue on the lower lip. Extraneous head movements were present with effort.

Oral kinaesthesia: Earlier speech therapy had focused on articulation to improve Maggie's oral kinaesthesia and the score in this area was close to normal.

Speech: Despite a good cleft palate repair and careful speech therapy management, she had very poor speech, marked by fluctuating hypernasality, dentalisation of lingual sounds and slow, breathy production of voice. Her inability to control saliva during speech meant that Maggie hardly opened her mouth when speaking. Her pre-eminent difficulty was that she was quite unable to produce rapid alternating speech movements in conversation. Although her weakness in the area of oral kinaesthesia had responded to therapy, her DDK, without lingual mobility, remained very poor and as a consequence so did her speech.

Emotional status: Maggie was a painfully shy and

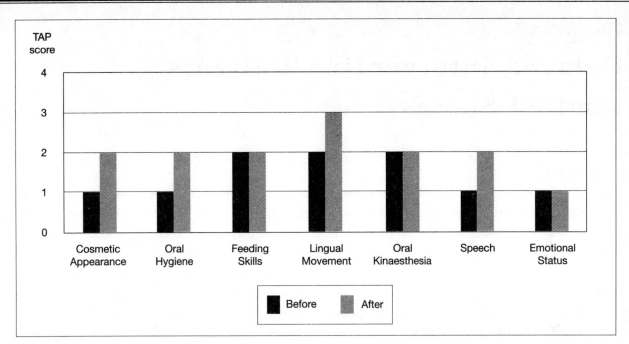

Figure 5
Comparison of total TAP scores before and after intervention

sensitive child who was very conscious of her speech problems.

Progress
The pre-operative total TAP score was 10.

Maggie's TAP results showed deficits in all areas considered as relevant in the assessment of tongue tie. Despite regular speech therapy which was geared to deal with the problems of cleft palate, speech remained poor because of an equally pertinent problem with tongue tie. Surgery was recommended and performed. This produced immediate improvement in movement, oral hygiene and speech.

However, due to the age at which surgery was performed, some problems connected with old incorrect speech habits remained. These would probably have responded to further therapy, but not surprisingly Maggie's motivation weakened,

and treatment lapsed. A common penalty of delayed surgical intervention is that the patient is disheartened by the thought of any prolongation of effort in speech therapy, and disillusioned when not 'cured' immediately after surgery.

When Maggie was discharged at her own request, a post-operative total TAP score of 14 was obtained.

Conclusions
Maggie was denied a simple and effective surgical option for an organic problem with tongue tie. This was because she also had a major deficit—a cleft palate—which took priority. The consequent delay in surgical treatment and prolongation of symptoms resulting from her tongue tie contributed to reduced expectation of improvement and subsequent curtailment of therapy, which had good potential for success.

Case History 5:

Delayed Intervention Delivers Limited Success

Hypothesis

Children over the age of 3 years usually need intensive speech therapy after surgery if they are to improve oral kinaesthesia and overcome undesirable speech habits.

History

Adam was 8 years old when seen in a pre-operative consultation for articulation difficulty. His father had an untreated tongue tie and very poor speech. Adam's tie had been noted at birth, but it was his dentist who recommended surgery. He had previously been assessed by two speech therapy clinics and had received therapy, but the tongue tie was not observed.

Observations

Cosmetic appearance: The tie was short, thick and tight on palpation. The tongue appeared small and flat, with a marked notch in the lingual margin. Adam had an open bite and breathed through his mouth.

Oral hygiene and dental health: Adam controlled excessive salivation produced during speech by maintaining a very small oral aperture and talking slowly.

Feeding skills: Adam was breastfed for 9 months and took solids well from 7 months of age, but could not lick.

Lingual movement: There was obvious impact on lingual movement: elevation of the tongue was not possible, but the tongue could be protruded a short way downwards and horizontally almost to the mucobuccal fold. Lateral movement produced concomitant head movement, limited retraction of the tongue was possible and circumlocution could be performed using the blade of the tongue. All movements requested required concentration and effort in their performance.

Oral kinaesthesia: Adam's previous experience of speech therapy had impacted on his oral kinaesthesia, which was only moderately impaired, and he could understand directional lingual movement. However, if unable to monitor his actions visually he could not produce repeated movements even at a slow rate of speed.

Speech: Adam's speech was very poor: his consonants were imprecise and he had involuntary pitch changes. Polysyllabic words and rapid speech were particularly challenging for him. He had acquired, and strongly developed, defensive habits of speech (including a pseudo-American accent with well-marked final R sounds) in his efforts to be understood. He spoke through clenched jaws so as to make articulatory contacts. At school, he was always being asked to repeat himself, and said he was 'sick of it'.

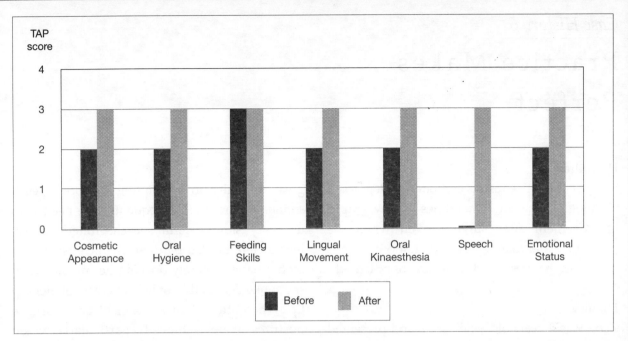

Figure 6

Comparison of total TAP scores before and after intervention

Emotional status: He presented as a quiet, determined little boy who was painfully aware of his difficulties. He went to a very competitive school and responded to his difficulties with pronunciation by using a small oral opening, and deliberately slow and careful speech. He had a tense manner, husky voice and a tight lower jaw.

Progress

Adam's pre-operative total TAP score was 13.

All critical areas of assessment were affected by lack of lingual mobility, and surgery was recommended. Following surgery, Adam had speech therapy in 3-month blocks for a year, during which time oral kinaesthesia, tongue movements, oral hygiene and confidence improved very slowly. However, speech was the last area to show improvement.

A post-operative total TAP score of 21 was obtained before discharge.

Conclusions

At the age of eight, Adam had acquired many habits of lingual movement, body language and speech which were maladaptations to his limitations of lingual movement. The improvements made after surgery and speech therapy required intensive effort. Maintaining these new habits requires concentration until mastery is reached. Although Adam achieved intelligibility he was not able to acquire spontaneity in speech before therapy was discontinued.

Case History 6:

Practice Makes Perfect

Hypothesis

Severe cumulative results of moderate degrees of ankyloglossia can sometimes show rapid improvement after surgery, even when the patient is older than 3 years, when motivation is high, and the prescribed exercises are practised.

History

Zena was 8 years old when seen, and presented with moderate disability in all seven areas of oromuscular function considered as criteria for surgery in cases of tongue tie.

Observations

Cosmetic appearance: The tongue tie was easily visible as a short, white membrane with traumatised thickenings from friction with the lower incisors. It was tight on palpation.

Oral hygiene and dental health: Poor lingual mobility affected oral hygiene: although tidy in all other respects, Zena was described as a 'messy eater' who could not get food off her teeth and developed a rash around her mouth from salivary residue.

Feeding skills: As a baby, Zena had been a slow feeder, cried a lot, and was felt to have been hungry and colicky. She was taken off the breast at 5 weeks, and she coped better with a bottle and on solids.

Lingual movement: Zena could localise and copy tongue movements correctly, but experienced great difficulty in attempting to copy speech sounds accurately. Consequently she needed to use very slow, careful speech. Tongue movements were limited by these characteristics, and by her habit of barely opening her mouth when she spoke. She could not lick ice cream off her top lip. When attempting assessment tasks, bizarre postures were achieved, particularly when attempting lateral movement.

Oral kinaesthesia: Zena had difficulty making the connection between speech sounds and tongue movements. She also found rapid utterance very difficult.

Speech: When she tried to speak loudly, her co-ordination would become quite disorganised. DDK was poor. Speech was often unintelligible, particularly under stresses such as speed, anxiety or excitement. Occasionally, she had difficulty even at conversational levels of speed. Zena habitually spoke slowly and carefully and interspersed her speech with 'um' and 'er'.

Emotional status: Zena presented as a shy, quiet, 'good' child. She was very aware of her tongue being 'different'.

Progress

The pre-operative total TAP score was 9.

The score on TAP was unexpectedly low, considering how well Zena presented at school and socially. Obviously she was coping by the

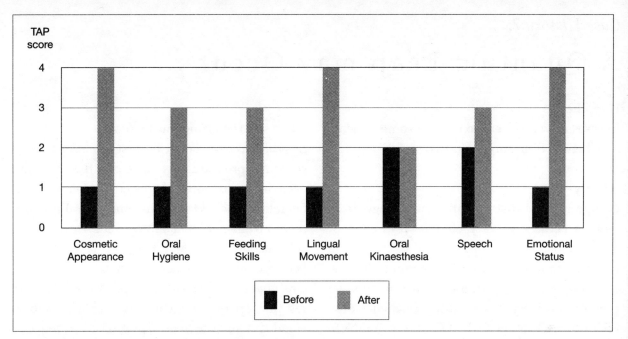

Figure 7

Comparison of total TAP scores before and after intervention

expenditure of considerable effort in activities demanding oromuscular co-ordination. Her parents were greatly relieved to hear that an operation could help Zena and surgery was arranged without delay. Zena was asked to practise a set of tongue exercises daily to assist in developing oral kinaesthetic sense and to increase her range of tongue movements. Initially, after surgery there was some concern as the expected improvements were slow to occur. It was then found that Zena had not persevered with her exercises pre or post-operatively!

The prescribed programme of speech exercises was instituted again, with good results, and 5 months after surgery Zena was found to have made great progress. She presented as giggly and talkative, had a full range of lingual movements at speed, and a nicely pointed tongue tip. She

was still making occasional articulation errors in rapid utterance, and was advised to continue with practice of the exercises set.

Zena obtained a total TAP score of 23 on discharge.

Conclusions

Excellent results were obtained in this case despite intervention being delayed to 8 years, possibly because of Zena's optimistic personality and the fact that strong habit factors had not been acquired. The improvement in the cosmetic appearance of the tongue was also a relief to this little girl. Zena's motivation was further enhanced by the relative ease with which she shed the bizarre movements she had been forced to make until surgery gave her greater freedom of lingual movement.

Case History 7:

A Quantum Leap may Occur ...

Hypothesis

In cases of very severe tongue tie some patients may benefit from surgery in two stages.

History

George had his first operation at the age of 18 months because of very obvious restriction of tongue movement and poverty of language. He had been communicating only in grunts and was obviously frustrated. After the first operation he acquired six very basic, mostly bilabial words (BOOM, BROOM, POO, BALL, MORE and NO). He was then referred to me for 3 months of speech therapy while progress was monitored.

Observations

Cosmetic appearance: George's tongue was large and wide, it was strongly indented in the midline and had no point. Narrowing of the tongue was observed when pointing strongly downwards, but no subtle changes of shape or position were observed. It was particularly difficult to see the underside of George's tongue since he could not elevate it, but the frenum felt tight on palpation.

Oral hygiene and dental health: George had never dribbled much, due probably to a habit of firm lip closure and very little vocal output. When first seen, he tended to have some food debris in, and the occasional rash around, his mouth. After his first operation he became a neat eater and wiped food off his mouth.

Feeding skills: George had been breastfed without difficulty for 8 months and was then weaned to the bottle. After surgery he began using the cup, sucked well from a straw and chewed better,

while still preferring mushy foods.

Lingual movement: Before his first operation George could not protrude the tongue past the vermilion even in the downward position. After his first operation he could pass the mucobuccal fold but made no other voluntary movement. Thus, he was still unable to elevate, retract, or make lateral or licking movements when assessed.

Oral kinaesthesia: When seen for assessment after his first operation, George was able to understand and attempt lingual protrusion on request; but although interested, he would not attempt other postures. After therapy he was more aware and used his fingers to help move his tongue to copy movements that he recognised but could not perform himself.

Speech: After therapy, George acquired 20 words but only used them after strong one-to-one stimulation. Often the words were unclear repetitions which would have seemed meaningless out of context. He did use 'Mama' and 'Dada' but many similar sounding vocalisations were used to cover a multitude of meanings. His voice was loud, deep and lacked inflection, as he always talked in a monotone.

Emotional status: A naturally assertive little boy, George was becoming negative and stubborn because of his very limited verbal output. He had a good understanding and showed a desire to communicate but was increasingly frustrated by his physical limitation.

Progress

When George was referred for a second operation

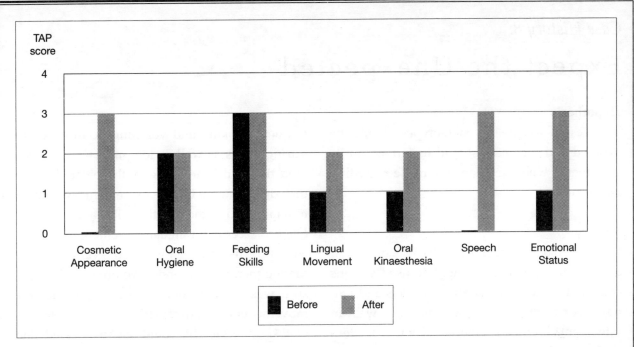

Figure 8

Comparison of total TAP scores before and after intervention

at 2 years his pre-operative total TAP score was 8.

Following the second operation, his progress was rapid. Slight post-operative discomfort was experienced. His mother noticed that he was having difficulty with certain sounds now being attempted spontaneously and further therapy was arranged.

George attended for four sessions during which he improved dramatically. He was acquiring five to six new words a week, and soon progressed to phrases. A language sample taken showed him using at least 71 single words and 42 phrases (some of three or more words) during one therapy session. He was even attempting consonant blends with modest success. Some pooling of saliva was noted with increasing volume of speech.

Benefits associated with the second operation were:

• His improved voice: the loud dysphonic

monotone had spontaneously normalised.

• His improved behaviour: reduction of stubbornness and negativity.

• His improved feeding: more efficient chewing and swallowing and lessened dribbling.

Four weeks after the second operation, his post-operative total TAP score was 18.

Conclusions

George had a very severe tongue tie, and in spite of early intervention—both therapeutic and surgical—continued to show symptoms of tongue tie. A second operation is then an appropriate option which provides the necessary lingual freedom, and the patient's progress then proceeds happily on the usual lines for children who have early intervention. This patient in fact showed very rapid progress once lingual freedom was achieved.

Case History 8:

Expect the Unexpected

Hypothesis

In cases of tongue tie, stereotypes should be avoided and each case should be judged on its own merits when decisions are made regarding intervention.

History

Janey, aged 3 years and 6 months, was described as 'essentially non-speaking'. She used various combinations of four nasalised vowels and two nasal consonants in six 'words'. She was an intelligent child with cerebral palsy whose identical twin had both mild cerebral palsy and tongue tie. There were major problems with muscle control because of her palsy, and feeding, speech and emotional reactions to stress were constant difficulties.

Observations

Cosmetic appearance: The tie was visible on retraction and extended to the lingual margin. When the involuntary tongue thrusting movements of her cerebral palsy occurred, the front of the tongue was tethered and pulled under by the tie.

Oral hygiene and dental health: This patient had constant and profuse dribbling, which was exacerbated by her habitual open-mouthed posture, and which often caused a rash around the mouth.

Feeding skills: Small bursts of lingual and labial activity were seen during eating. Janey could suck strongly from a straw, and dealt with solids with a combined chewing and sucking motion. Swallowing was performed with lips apart and the tongue thrusting. She gagged easily and frequent choking and vomiting occurred daily, during meals as well as long afterwards, when food that had been stuck on the palate became dislodged. Lateral tongue movements were used to retain food in the mouth while eating.

Lingual movement: Lingual movement was limited to protrusion to just within the vermilion, the tongue then curling under. Voluntary labial closure was possible on request, but no tongue movements were attempted.

Oral kinaesthesia: This could not be assessed, and Janey refused to attempt any tasks outside her scope.

Speech: Janey would attempt to communicate with vocalising and facial expression but was unintelligible to those who did not know her code. She was reported to have recently reduced her volume of speech, and now used only seven poorly pronounced words.

Emotional status: This intelligent child was forced into a babyish and regressed posture by her physical limitations. She reacted by controlling her environment with a habit of catastrophic reaction to stress, and cried uncontrollably for seemingly minor causes. Janey received much stimulation from her devoted family and her receptive language was good.

Progress

Janey's pre-operative total TAP score was 3.

Her cerebral palsy made the decision to operate a difficult one and her parents made the final choice hoping for improved eating habits. In the

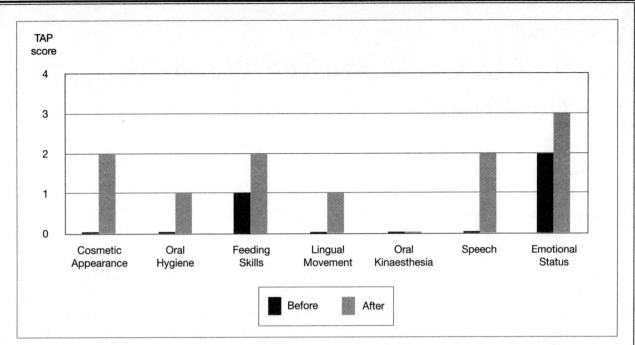

Figure 9

Comparison of total TAP scores before and after intervention

event, Janey responded well to surgery, with early improvements in feeding, reduction of dribbling, improved lip closure, and significantly, increased willingness to attempt words. Lingual movements increased in range and were better controlled, and involuntary elevation of the tongue to the upper lip was seen. Dribbling reduced, though splashing still occurred with effort.

At discharge, she was using long sentences, although control of pronunciation, voice, breathing and salivation remained erratic. Improvement in feeding skills, emotional status and communication were the main benefits from surgery. The small but very significant improvement in her score following surgery represented a massive change in Janey's abilities, and she became able to control her volatile emotions by verbalising them in socially acceptable ways. Her

expressive language changed to the point where she was using speech spontaneously to tell stories, ask questions, express feelings, control her environment and even to tell jokes! She attended for therapy at intervals over a 5 year period. Her post-operative total TAP score was 11.

Conclusions

Recommending surgery for tongue tie in a patient with cerebral palsy or other serious disorder would appear to be a radical action, and all implications should be carefully studied. In this case conventional therapy had been tried for several years with little progress, and Janey's parents decided that the operation represented a valid and hopeful option. The decision was a fortunate one, and she made gains that would not have been achieved otherwise.

Case History 9:

When You Can't See the Wood for the Trees

Hypothesis

Some cases present with so much symptomatology that a differential diagnosis becomes very complex, and the surest clue to a diagnosis is the simple physical one, of seeing and palpating the tie.

History

Jason, aged 6 years, had been having speech therapy from the age of 2 years and 6 months, with little improvement. Multiple difficulties in infancy included sleep problems, projectile vomiting and diarrhoea, presumed lactose intolerance and constant screaming up until 10 months old. At 6 years, he still had enuresis and was encopretic, preferred eating soft foods and showed regressed behaviour. There was a family history of tongue tie.

Observations

Cosmetic appearance: The tongue looked small, and the fan-shaped tie ran across the floor of the mouth and ended at the base of the lower front teeth.

Oral hygiene and dental health: Hyper-salivation during lengthy utterance was noted. Jason had dribbled profusely when younger.

Feeding skills: Jason had a long history of feeding problems. His mother had mastitis frequently while breastfeeding Jason, and at five months the infant still required breastfeeding every two to three hours, right through the day and night. Poor co-ordination of sucking and swallowing may have contributed to his digestive problems of projectile vomiting and evacuation. He was weaned at 12 months, but remained a slow and fussy eater, with poor skills in chewing and licking. He drank often to facilitate swallowing. He chose softer foods and could manage these without a drink, liked bread but found rolls too bulky to chew, and was described as a 'messy eater'.

Lingual movement: Limited lingual movement was possible, most positions being achieved by trial and error and accompanied by shakiness and blinking. He was unable to elevate the tongue and needed to grip it between his teeth to achieve horizontal protrusion, even then only reaching up to the vermilion.

Oral kinaesthesia: Poor DDK and oral kinaesthesia were noted. Jason was unable to co-ordinate more than one consonant at moderate speed, and was unable to copy any tongue positions without watching himself in a mirror.

Speech: Jason used such a simple vocabulary that at one stage of his previous speech therapy pro-

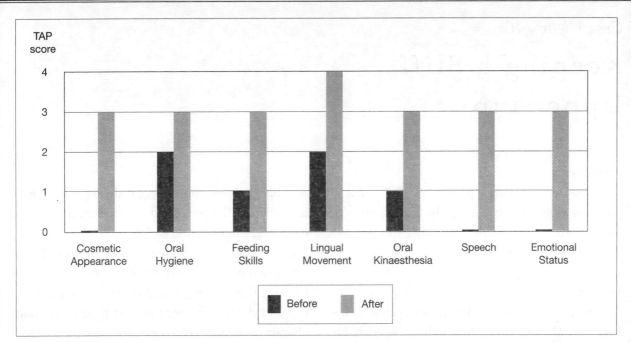

Figure 10

Comparison of total TAP scores before and after intervention

gramme he was thought to be language disabled. He was inaccurate in his pronunciation of vowels, consonants and their blends in conversation. Inconsistent errors were a feature of his speech; however, many consonants could be elicited in single words or with stimulation.

Emotional Status: Jason presented as a happy-go-lucky, dependent child. He ignored his speech problems as he ignored physical signals indicating a need for toileting.

Progress

The pre-operative total TAP score was 6.

Following surgery, steady improvement took place in speech and feeding, and also became apparent in more age-appropriate, boyish and independent behaviour. However, old habits of dependency had been well entrenched, and these were not eradicated without a struggle. As his school work improved, he became an achiever and shot ahead, particularly in his reading skills. It was hoped that with increasing maturation, motivation for continence would also emerge. He was discharged after 12 months of therapy with clear speech and a post-operative assessment score of 22.

Case History 10:

Keeping a Stiff Upper Lip

Hypothesis

The idea that ignoring a problem will cause it to go away does not always apply, and in cases of tongue tie, may cause prolongation of the patient's discomfort.

History

Patient Frank was self-referred and came to me because of his dissatisfaction with his speech. He was 29 years old and his work involved daily lecturing. His frequent errors of pronunciation and inability to control salivation during prolonged speech caused inattention and attracted criticism from his audience, and he described himself as 'becoming paranoid' about his speech. There was a family history of tongue tie, but his tight frenum had been thought to be too mild for surgery.

Observations

Cosmetic appearance: The tongue was notched at the margin, wide and deeply grooved in the midline where it was pulled down by the tie. The tie was best seen in retraction when it looked thin and was deeply sunk in the lingual tissue. It was tight on palpation.

Oral hygiene and dental health: The patient described his tongue as 'always sloppy'. Oral hygiene was a major preoccupation for this patient, who was conscious of salivary profusion and had trouble controlling it during his lecturing. His dentist remarked on food stains on his teeth and many dental caries.

Feeding skills: Frank preferred finely cut meat and Chinese food because of the relative ease of masticating them. He washed down his food with copious drinks and was unable to lick. He had always bitten ice cream or rubbed it on the blade of the tongue.

Lingual movement: Horizontal protrusion of the tongue was possible only up to the mucobuccal fold. All lingual movements requested in assessment could be performed, although hesitantly. Thus, limitation of movement was not severe.

Oral kinaesthesia: The patient needed explanations and a visual model to attempt movements requested for assessment. Control of pitch and articulation varied involuntarily when Frank experienced stress. So although lingual movement was adequate for giving the patient access to articulatory positions, poor oral kinaesthesia was a significant limiting factor.

Speech: Frank had difficulty pronouncing polysyllabic words and certain consonants. He was often forced to look for alternative words because of pronunciation difficulty. This was a constant problem in the professional arena when he might be forced to use a technical term for

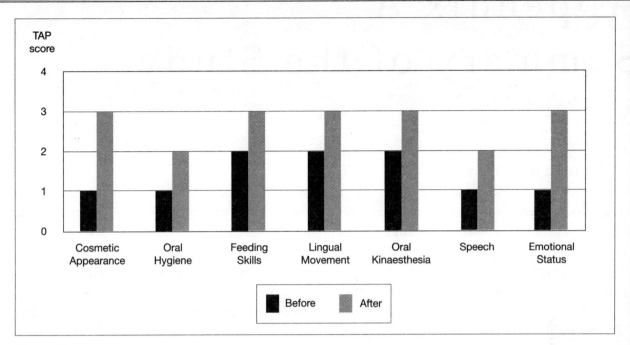

TAP score

Figure 11

Comparison of total TAP scores before and after intervention

which there was no substitute. He frequently suffered from sore throats because of his habit of tense, dysphonic vocalisation.

Emotional status: The long term problems he experienced had affected Frank's self esteem, and caused constant anxiety. He was required to present confidently in his chosen profession but his confidence in his abilities was undermined by his poor communication skills.

Progress

The pre-operative total TAP score was 10.

Surgery was recommended and took place and recovery was uneventful. Unlike several other adult clients Frank noted very little discomfort following surgery. Subsequently he attended for several months of therapy. Steady improvement was noted in all areas, particularly oral hygiene, speech and self confidence.

Due to various circumstances, Frank decided to terminate therapy sooner than was advised. In view of his delayed surgery, Frank was advised to continue to practise his exercises so as to counter habits of incorrect speech production. Frank was discharged with a post-operative total TAP score of 19.

Conclusions

Several years later, Frank returned for therapy, to improve problems with articulation, voice rhythm and confidence regarding his speech. With determination and regular practice we were able to address issues which had not been fully dealt with earlier.

Appendix A
Summary of the Study

INTRODUCTION

Between 1981 and 1982, the author carried out a study of 17 patients with tongue tie who were referred to the Speech Therapy department of the Children's Hospital (Royal Alexandra Hospital for Children) at Camperdown in Sydney for assessment, with a query regarding possible aetiology of tongue tie.

Following this short study, the author continued to document all cases of tongue tie referred to her. Of the 1,290 patients referred for speech therapy between October 1981 and October 1997, 256 were perceived as requiring assessment for tongue tie. These patients were assessed by means of a protocol developed by the author. Two hundred patients with complete records were included in the study. It is these patients with complete records who constitute the subjects of the study.

OBJECTIVES
- To determine whether tongue tie was a problem which had a real impact on the development and production of speech.
- To devise an assessment and treatment plan.
- To draw conclusions about the usefulness of surgical release of the frenum.

METHODOLOGY

Data were collected on 200 patients who were referred to the author for assessment or speech therapy, or both, and who were found to have limited tongue movement and an abnormal frenum. Some patients (139) were referred because tongue tie had been suspected; the remainder were referred for speech therapy, and during assessment were found to have a tongue tie. More subjects (119) in the study were drawn from the author's private practice than through the public hospital system (81). Although initially there were more hospital patients, they tended to move away from the area or to fail to attend, hence their records were incomplete.

Each patient was assessed on the basis of seven criteria, which covered appearance, function and speech. These were cosmetic appearance, oral hygiene and dental health, feeding skills, lingual movement, oral kinaesthesia, speech and emotional status. Depending on the results obtained, speech therapy or surgery with post-operative speech therapy, or both, were recommended. The same seven-criteria method of assessment, the Tongue tie Assessment Protocol (or TAP), was then used to monitor progress.

RESULTS

A total of 200 patients (150 male, 50 female) were assessed by means of TAP. Of these, 86 (43%) had a family history of tongue tie and 45 (23%) had more than one family member known to have the same condition. The age range was from 3 months to 29 years. Only two patients were over the age of 18 years. The age breakdown is detailed in Table A1.

Table A1
Age breakdown

Age	No. of patients
1 year and under	15
Over 1 year and under 4 years	59
Over 4 years and under 10 years	111
Over 10 years	15
Total	200

A breakdown of assessment findings for the 200 patients is shown in Table A2.

Table A2
Assessment findings

Characteristic	No. of patients
Delayed or defective speech	200
One type of speech defect	146
Two types of speech defects	47
Three types of speech defects	7
Secondary emotional disorder	152
Poor oral hygiene and dental health	67
History of feeding difficulty	40
Congenital abnormality (e.g. cleft palate, cerebral palsy, developmental delay)	29
Hearing problems and ear infections	23
Prone to respiratory infections	17

Of the 200 subjects in the study, 139 were referred specifically because they had been identified as possibly having tongue tie. Others were discovered as a result of requests for speech therapy. Surgery was recommended for 196 patients. Of these, 175 were operated upon and were followed-up after surgery.

All of the patients showed an improvement in speech after surgery and, where indicated, task-specific speech therapy. The rate of improvement was slower for the older patients. Twelve patients required the operation to be performed in two stages.

All patients showed a whitish appearance under the tongue in the first week after surgery. As healing took place the whitish appearance faded gradually. Most patients whose ties extended to the lingual margin continued to show lingual notching after the operation with no diminution of function. One patient was observed to have reduced notching after surgery.

When the simple exercises devised for use after surgery were practised regularly, patients made good progress. However, progress depended on the age of the patient at the time of operation—children under three generally acquired normal speech and lingual function without prolonged therapy. Older subjects required from 3 months to a year of therapy, depending on factors such as age, motivation and the presence of other disabilities or emotional problems. Patients with feeding difficulties, dribbling, open-mouthed posture and tongue thrust often required prolonged therapy.

CONCLUSIONS

Tongue tie was found to have a significant effect not only on the development and production of speech but also on behaviour and appearance. Surgical intervention combined with appropriate speech therapy was found to be very effective in treating tongue tie. The assessment protocol devised, TAP, was found to be a reliable indicator for deciding whether surgical intervention was appropriate and for quantifying the improvement after treatment.

Appendix B
Assessing Ankyloglossia

INTRODUCTION

This appendix gives instructions for carrying out an assessment on a patient with suspected ankyloglossia or tongue tie, using the Tongue tie Assessment Protocol (TAP) described in Chapter 4.

The assessment is carried out under seven headings. For each heading, a score is given using the scoring criteria provided and notes are made of significant findings. Page 70 contains an example of a completed form, which includes the scores obtained as well as the significant findings noted. This form may constitute the reporting mechanism at an initial interview and at subsequent reviews. Page 71 contains a blank form which may be copied and used without infringing copyright.

CASE HISTORY

A skilfully taken history will provide additional details about all areas of the assessment field and is an essential part of the assessment. In particular, feeding and emotional factors will be most appropriately enlarged upon during history taking. Familiarity with the characteristic problems of tongue tie allows the speech pathologist to elicit significant information the parent may not have felt to be relevant. Children's fears may be eased by their listening to the case history being taken, as they often feel relief when hearing that their symptoms are recognised and understood.

COSMETIC APPEARANCE

The appearance of the tongue at rest and during activity should be noted. Any grooving on the dorsal lingual surface, notching of the lingual margin or dimpling of the tongue on elevation should be noted as it could signify tongue tie. The frenum must be viewed and if possible, palpated. The extent, thickness and appearance of the frenum should be noted. Pain on movement must also be noted, as it is not normal and could be due to the tightness of the frenum.

Table B1
Scoring cosmetic appearance

Finding	Score
The frenum and tongue are conspicuously different at rest and during movement	0
The frenum is tight, and there is obvious abnormal movement	1
The frenum is visible during speech and is tight on palpation	2
The frenum is visible during speech but is not tight	3
The tongue has a normal appearance, pointed tip and intact lingual margin	4

ORAL HYGIENE AND DENTAL HEALTH

The mouth should be checked for dental caries, healthiness of soft tissue and food debris in and around the lips. Special note should be made of the patient's ability to control saliva during speech. Problems with dribbling or splashing saliva, or a rash caused by excess saliva wetting the area around the lips should be noted. A history of dental visits made by the patient should be obtained and compared with the dental history of siblings. If the mother is still responsible for the child's dental hygiene this should be noted, as it may mask a latent problem. The patient's bite should also be observed, as malocclusions are often found in patients with tongue tie.

For older patients, the ability to suck, swallow, lick, chew or cope with bulky food needs to be noted. Special arrangements that may be in use to make feeding easier (such as drinks to accompany food, pureeing foods, or providing special diets) should be noted. The history of early feeding habits should relate particularly to co-ordination of oral musculature under pressure as with large mouthfuls or in conditions of haste.

Besides obtaining information from the parent or patient, it would be useful to observe current eating habits.

Table B2
Scoring oral hygiene and dental health

Finding	Score
There are dental caries, food debris, a bitten tongue, a rash and frequent dribble	0
There are dental caries, food debris, rash and dribbling	1
There are dental caries, or dribbling and rash around the lips	2
There is hypersalivation during rapid speech and occasional dribble	3
There are no current problems or history of excessive dribbling	4

Table B3
Scoring feeding skills

Finding	Score
Current breastfeeding problems, or other severe persistent feeding problems still apparent	0
Slow, fussy feeding, poor chewing and licking, drinking during meals to facilitate swallowing	1
Slow eating of all foods, and inability to lick	2
Problems in infancy but none now	3
No problems at any stage	4

FEEDING SKILLS
The assessment of feeding skills should commence with questions about any maternal discomfort during breastfeeding, a history of mastitis, cracked, sore or bleeding nipples, as well as any difficulty the infant may have had in achieving latch-on, sucking, or coping with the flow of milk.

LINGUAL MOVEMENT
Lingual proficiency is assessed by asking the patient to adopt various tongue positions. Some patients may require the position to be demonstrated while others may only be able to accomplish the movement in front of a mirror. Either case may imply poor oral kinaesthesia and should

therefore be noted. The patient should be asked to perform the following six tasks and a score determined in accordance with Table B4 and the number of tasks successfully completed.

Table B4
Scoring for lingual movement

Finding	Score
1 task achieved	0
2 tasks achieved	1
3 tasks achieved	2
4 tasks achieved	3
5 or 6 tasks achieved	4

Task 1. Protrusion with downward pointing
On requesting protrusion with downward pointing, the quickness of response and distance protruded should be noted. It should also be noted whether the tongue passes the mucobuccal fold and the vermilion and remains steady in this position. Curling of the sides of the tongue or the presence of excess saliva are also important signs and should be noted. This task should be regarded as completed if the tongue can be protruded downwards and held steady for five seconds with no difficulty.

Task 2. Horizontal protrusion
On requesting horizontal protrusion in the midline, the speed of production of this movement should be compared with that of downward protrusion. In patients with tongue tie, the distance reached is usually less, and the tongue is able to maintain the position only momentarily. If the tongue can be protruded past the vermilion with-

out being supported on the lower lip, this task can be regarded as completed.

Task 3. Protrusion with upward pointing
On requesting protrusion with upward pointing, independent elevation of the tongue towards the upper lip will nearly always be found to be impossible in patients with tongue tie. Features of the attempt, such as compensatory or guiding movements of the head, lips or eyes should be noted. The sides of the tongue will often be more active than the tip or middle, causing the frenum to appear as a thin, broad and flattened structure, sometimes showing a minimal tip. Most patients with tongue tie will avoid this movement and be aware that they cannot perform it. Free elevation of the tongue past the upper lip and with the mouth open can be regarded as successful completion of this task.

Task 4. Circumlocution
Circumlocution may be explained to the patient as the action required for licking ice cream off the lips and all around the mouth. Features of response to be noted include whether the teeth are being used to hold the tongue in position and whether the mouth is open or shut. The task can be regarded as having been completed if there is a smooth circular movement of the tongue around the mouth. If the tongue is supported on the lower lip, or the lower lip or the blade of the tongue is used to rub the upper lip, the task cannot be regarded as having been completed.

Task 5. Lateral movement
When requesting lateral movement, note grading of effort and its consequence—controlled or uncontrolled movement. Smooth and accurate movement from left to right can be regarded as successfully completing this task. Any inaccuracy, deterioration of movement at speed or tendency

to move the jaw or head to assist in continuous right/left movements should be recorded.

Task 6. Retraction of the tongue

When requesting retraction it may be useful to instruct the patient to 'push the tongue as far back as possible' and observe results. If the movement cannot be elicited voluntarily, yawning may be requested. If the patient is an infant, it is often possible to observe while crying, laughing, or making palatal clicks.

Where the patient is observed to have difficulty performing the tasks, visual clues such as using a mirror to monitor actions or watching the speech pathologist demonstrate the task, may be given. If visual clues had to be given, this should be noted.

It is particularly important to note poverty of movement, which leads the patient to reiterate the few movements he or she can produce, even if they are irrelevant to the task.

If the patient is able to retract the tongue to show the frenum, the task has been successfully completed.

ORAL KINAESTHESIA

Standard speech therapy techniques may be used to check oral kinaesthesia. The same tasks cannot be used for all patients because of age differences. The assessment is carried out in two parts (see below). A score is given for each part and the average of the two scores is taken as the overall score for oral kinaesthesia.

Children under the age of two cannot be assessed for oral kinaesthesia and should be given a score of 0.

With very young children (between 2 and 3 years) it is possible to ask them to copy smiling, poking the tongue out, filling cheeks with air and popping them, alternating smiling and pouting, Skippy noises and nonsense syllables, and thus to obtain an impression of their kinaesthetic level.

These are activities which children with normal oral function would perform in play. When scoring, allocate a score between 0 and 4 in proportion to how well the tasks were performed.

Children over 3 years and all other patients can be scored using the following procedures.

Part 1. Test of diadochokinetic syllable rate

The ability to coordinate 1, 2, and 3 consonants with a neutral vowel in slow and fast repetitions is used to judge diadochokinesis. 'Slow' repetition is considered as 1 repetition per second, and 'fast' repetitions as 4 repetitions per second. The therapist may count the repetitions or demonstrate the task if needed.

Table B5

Part 1. Scoring oral kinaesthesia

Finding	Score
Able to coordinate 1 consonant only in 10 slow repetitions	0
Able to coordinate 1 consonant in 10 fast repetitions	1
Able to coordinate 2 consonants together in 10 slow repetitions	2
Able to coordinate 2 consonants together in 15 fast repetitions	3
Able to coordinate 3 consonants together in 15 fast repetitions	4

Part 2. Performing required tasks

Where the patient is under 5 years, the tasks given in Table B6 can be demonstrated. Otherwise, the task should be described to the patient who should then perform it.

Table B6
Tasks to be performed

Task	Under 5 yrs	Over 5 yrs
Hold air in the cheeks and pop	Once	3 times
Protrude the tongue in the midline, withdraw and protrude to the right, withdraw, and protrude to the left	Once	3 times
Protrude and make a cross on the lips with the tongue	Omit	3 times
Protrude and make an inclined cross (X) on the lips	Omit	3 times
Poke tongue into left cheek, out at middle of lips, and into right cheek	Omit	3 times

A score should be given in accordance with Table B7. For patients under 5 years, an additional 3 points should be added.

Table B7
Part 2. Scoring for tasks performed

Finding	Score
1 task achieved	0
2 tasks achieved	1
3 tasks achieved	2
4 tasks achieved	3
5 tasks achieved	4

Add the scores recorded for Part 1 (Table B5) and Part 2 (Table B7) and divide by 2. The result is the score for oral kinaesthesia.

SPEECH
An age-appropriate articulation test that incorporates assessment of connected speech and rapid, loud and whispered utterances should be used. It is important to note phrasing, voice quality and the length of sentences in spontaneous speech. All these aspects of speech may be altered in a patient who is having difficulty manipulating his or her tongue because of limited mobility, poor coordination and lack of precision of movement. Consistency of speech attempts under different conditions of speed, volume or prolonged utterance must also be recorded. Based on the results obtained, a score should be allocated in accordance with Table B8.

Table B8
Scoring for speech

Finding	Score
Severely defective, or disorders in 3 modes (articulation, voice, resonance, fluency or rhythm) or more	0
Moderate speech disorder in 2 modes	1
Mildly defective in the articulatory mode only	2
Within normal limits with a few inconsistencies	3
Normal speech at all times	4

EMOTIONAL STATUS
Observation of patients and parental descriptions

will give the speech pathologist many clues as to the patients' feelings about their condition, and their emotional status in general. It will also be useful to observe the way in which responses are made to the tasks that had to be performed above. A score should be allocated in accordance with the appropriate finding given in Table B9.

Table B9
Scoring for emotional status

Finding	Score
Difficult to manage and has more than one symptom of behavioural disturbance	0
Upset by failures during testing and has one symptom of behavioural disturbance	1
Upset by failures in testing, speech or lingual difficulties	2
Confident in all areas but sensitive about lingual difficulties	3
Confident and stable with no emotional or behavioural problems	4

TOTAL SCORE

Add the scores obtained on each of the seven criteria of the TAP. **If a tie is present and the total score is 15 or less, a conclusion can be made that surgery is warranted.**

Surgery may also be warranted for older patients, or for those who have had prolonged therapy previously, who may score highly in one area and thus elevate the total score to over 15 while still demonstrating significant deficits. Such patients achieve very good results after surgery.

The same seven criteria on the TAP should be used to evaluate improvement at follow-up visits.

Example of a Tongue Tie Assessment

TONGUE TIE ASSESSMENT
using the Tongue tie Assessment Protocol (TAP)

Name:	John Macdonald	Date of Birth:	10–10–90
Address:	10 Riverside Place, Seaforth NSW 2112		
Telephone:	(02) 8987 6543	Date Seen:	15-05–97

Criterion	Score*	Comments
Cosmetic Appearance	2	Marked indentation of the lingual margin with strong grooving in the midline. The short tie can be felt on gentle palpation, but can only be seen during speech movements, as John cannot elevate his tongue freely.
Oral Hygiene and Dental Health	3	Profuse dribbling in babyhood. Now, John wipes his lips often. There is evidence of salivary profusion during rapid utterance. Several dental caries noted.
Feeding Skills	2	John could not be breastfed, because his mother developed mastitis, but he fed well on the bottle. Currently he eats solids very quickly but does not chew well, swallowing lumps whole. He facilitates swallowing with drinking. Frequent ear infections from 12 months, and grommets inserted at 4 years.
Lingual Movement	1	John is unable to lick his lips but makes brief, poorly controlled lateral movements. Elevation of the tongue is not possible. Protrusion is only possible up to the vermilion. Circumlocution is only possible inside the lips. The tie is visible on involuntary retraction of the tongue.
Oral Kinaesthesia	0	Very poor. John is unable to make lingual postures unless watching himself in a mirror. Lip movements can be made. He refuses to attempt tasks involving rapid speech, will only count slowly to 5, though he knows his numbers. Coordination of speech and breathing is poor, he can only repeat 1 consonant slowly, 10 times.
Speech	0	His speech is disturbed in 3 aspects, resonance, articulation and rhythm. Speech is jerky, can be both husky and nasal in tone and consonants are mispronounced. He is often barely audible and unintelligible. Family history of tongue tie.
Emotional Status	1	John has very little confidence and there is sibling rivalry with verbose brothers. He is dependent and demanding and complains frequently. He appears to be aware of his limited lingual mobility. He responds well to individual attention.
Total score	9	

*Key: 0 = Severe problem; 1 = Moderately severe problem; 2 = Mild problem; 3 = Within normal limits; 4 = Above average

RECOMMENDATIONS:

This total score indicates that John will benefit from surgery. He has been given exercises for enhancing oral kinaesthesia and articulation therapy will be commenced while his parents consider the option to have surgery to free the tongue. I feel that he will benefit in all areas of speech and behaviour with appropriate intervention, provided it is not unduly delayed.

TONGUE TIE ASSESSMENT
using the Tongue tie Assessment Protocol (TAP)

Name:		Date of Birth:	
Address:			
Telephone:		Date Seen:	

Criterion	Score*	Comments
Cosmetic Appearance		
Oral Hygiene and Dental Health		
Feeding Skills		
Lingual Movement		
Oral Kinaesthesia		
Speech		
Emotional Status		
Total score		

*Key: 0 = Severe problem; 1 = Moderately severe problem; 2 = Mild problem; 3 = Within normal limits; 4 = Above average

RECOMMENDATIONS:

(This form reproduced from *Tongue Tie—from confusion to clarity* by Carmen Fernando)

Appendix C
Surgical Procedures

The following techniques are employed in the surgical release of tongue tie by Doctors Edward Beckenham, Martin Glasson and Hugh Martin:

BECKENHAM METHOD

Under general anaesthetic, with the patient intubated, the tongue tip is lifted forward and the tongue tie placed on the stretch with sharp scissors dissection. The tight band is dissected until the base of the tongue is reached, and any tight fibres are divided. This usually leads to a separation at the floor of the mouth between the papillae of the submandibular ducts.

At that point, a cat gut suture is placed between the mucosal layers and possibly up the undersurface of the tongue to close the mucosal space.

The patient is admitted as a day–stay and complications are extremely uncommon.

GLASSON METHOD

Induction of anaesthesia may utilise the intravenous route or inhalation, depending upon the preferences of the anaesthetist. Maintenance of the airway during the operation can be with an endotracheal tube, or a nasopharyngeal tube. The nasopharyngeal tube is used for most patients as it is less invasive and surgeon and anaesthetist do not have to compete for access to the mouth.

The frenum linguae is **divided transversely** using cutting diathermy. It is important that a protective guard cover all but about 1 cm of the diathermy tip, and this ensures that the lower lip is not exposed to the risk of accidental burning. Having divided the avascular frenum, the transverse incision then extends into the tongue musculature (genioglossus) for a sufficient depth to achieve maximum release. Just how far to go is a matter of surgical judgement, and it is felt that this aspect of the operation is the single most important aspect which ensures a good result.

Having released the tongue in this manner, the final step is to suture the mucosa **longitudinally** with interrupted 4/0 cat gut sutures. It is very important to include **mucosa only** in the sutures; the muscle fibres which have been divided are not included in the closure but become covered by mucosa.

Needless to say, the anaesthetic does not involve muscular paralysis so that the patient wakes up very quickly following completion of the procedure. Some patients experience brief distress in the recovery room but oral Panadol usually suffices for analgesia.

It is perfectly safe for the patient to immediately resume normal oral intake, and many patients report visiting Macdonald's on their way home! However, moderation is advised!

MARTIN METHOD

A clamp is applied to the frenulum when the patient is anaesthetised deeply enough to be able to remove the mask for a short time, after which the anaesthetic mask is replaced for 3 or 4 minutes. The clamp must include the whole frenulum so that complete division is achieved. Care must be taken to avoid the orifices of the submandibular ducts.

The mask is then removed, and the crushed, devascularised area is divided with fine pointed scissors. Occasionally, if the frenulum is extremely short, the view of the area is insufficient to allow adequate placement of the clamp, so a second application is necessary.

With this method there is no bleeding and no need for sutures. On rare occasions the reapplication of the anaesthetic mask displaces the clamp laterally and causes tearing of the frenulum. If this occurs the surgeon must be prepared to effect haemostasis either by suture or by diathermy.

This method also avoids endotracheal intubation and is felt to be a less invasive anaesthetic technique. Pain is minimal with this method.

Appendix D
Exercises for Improving Lingual Proficiency

This appendix contains exercises which can be used to enhance sensory and motor aspects of oromuscular function with patients both before and after surgery. The exercises are in two sections—one for children and one for adults. The drawing of a section of the oral cavity given in Figure D1 may be used to supplement visual clues the patient receives from doing the exercises in front of a mirror and may be used with both child and adult patients.

Figure D1
Section of Oral Cavity

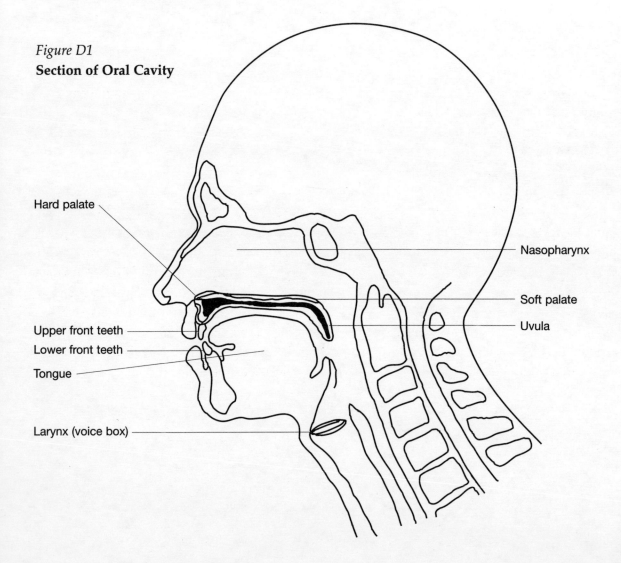

Hard palate

Nasopharynx

Soft palate

Uvula

Upper front teeth

Lower front teeth

Tongue

Larynx (voice box)

EXERCISES FOR CHILDREN

These exercises aim to enlarge the scope of tongue movements in young children by promoting oro-muscular movements in a play situation while focussing on both visual and tactile sensory feedback.

Circumlocution

- Draw a circle around the child's mouth with your finger, and ask him or her to try to follow your finger with his or her tongue. This can be called a 'race' or a tracking game.
- Draw another circle, using different textures, substances and tastes. The aim is to increase lingual sensitivity and interest in the use of the tongue in licking. You might choose Vegemite, honey, jam, ice cream, an iced block, or an ice cube. Ask the child to guess what you are using with eyes closed, and describe it as hot, cold, sticky, or runny. Now introduce new words to describe it. Next ask the child to lick around the mouth to remove the stimulus.

Protrusion

- While looking in a mirror, the child is asked to point the tongue at a target held in front of him. By pointing as hard as he can, a narrowed tongue with a tip will be achieved.
- Move the target by raising, lowering or shifting to left and right and ask the child to point to it. Acknowledge each effort and reward as appropriate.

Elevation

- Ask the child to bite his or her teeth lightly, and hold the posture while putting a smear of acceptable food (honey or Vegemite) on the upper lip. Ask the child to lick it off, opening the mouth very slowly while the tongue is elevated. Demonstrate.
- Touch the alveolar ridge behind the incisors with edible stimuli and ask the child to press the tongue against it and keep the stimulus in place. A piece of cheese or a sultana may be used. Later, the child may try to open the lips slowly, while keeping the tongue elevated.

Retraction

- Yawning produces a highly retracted tongue movement. Ask the child to yawn while watching himself in the mirror. Talk about the movement. Demonstrating an exaggerated yawn often stimulates the child to imitate quite naturally.

Exercises for lingual mobility and developing oral kinaesthesia can also be practised in play with the 'Mr Tongue' story, which follows. The speech pathologist or parent who is reading the story can point to the relevant portion of the drawing in *Figure D1* (to identify the part of the oral musculature referred to), or to the appropriate movement illustrated in Plates 25-31. The child sits facing a mirror so that movements may be monitored and compared at need with those of the adult who sits behind, also facing the mirror.

'Mr. Tongue' Story

Mr Tongue lives in a round pink house.
(the adult and the child point to the child's mouth)
This house is soft and pink and slippery, and just the right kind and size. Mr Tongue has a front door,
(point to the child's lips)
which is called the **Lips,** and a back door which is called the **Throat.**
(point to the child's throat)
The walls of the house are called the **Cheeks.** The ceiling of his house is called the **Palate.**
(point to the drawing in Figure D1 showing the line of the palate)
Under the roof is an upstairs room called the **Nose,**
(point to the nasal cavity)
but nobody goes there. When the front door is open you can see a fence, which is made of **Teeth.**
(point to the child's teeth)

There are two rows of teeth: **Top Teeth** and **Bottom Teeth.** Sometimes, old teeth fall out, and new ones grow in their place.

Mr Tongue is happy in his very own house. He is busy too. He says words, he sings songs, he plays tricks and slips and slides and makes faces or noises, and sometimes he rests when he is tired. He has work to do when you eat, or drink, or talk.

Here is Mr Tongue in his house, with his back door, his front door, that opens and closes and his fences.
(point to each named part of the mouth)

Now, let's read a Mr Tongue story, and you can do the actions.

Mr Tongue was curled up small in his bed, asleep. Then he woke up. He stretched
(point to Plate 25)

He reached up to the roof of his house ,
(point to Plate 26)

and he pushed against the walls
(push your tongue against your cheeks)
then he curled up small again. Then he thought, 'I'm lonely. I will go for a walk, I might meet some friends.' So, up he got.

He opened the gate
(your lips open)
he went past the fence
(point to Plate 27)

he looked to the left
(go to the left side of your mouth, point to Plate 28)

then he looked to the right.
(go to the right, point to Plate 29)

Then he chose the middle road. Out he went. He tried to go up the road.
(point to Plate 30, try to reach as far as you can, it might be difficult, but can you do it?)

Then he went down the road.
(point to Plate 31)
What do you think he saw?

He looked up at the sky. It was a sunny day. He saw a see-saw. It went up and down.
'I can do that too,' he said. He put a little square of white paper on his tongue.
(Place a small square of paper on the tip of the child's tongue)

Then he moved his tongue up and down, three times. When he was tired he went inside his house and rested. When he felt strong again, he came out.

Mr Tongue saw a cat walking on the fence. What a clever cat! It didn't fall off. Mr Tongue wanted to try. He got on the fence very carefully.
(Touch the bottom row of teeth with your tongue.)
He balanced on the fence and walked, all along to the end. Can you do it? He fell off! But he did it again.

He even tried the other fence, the top one. Can you do it?
(Touch the top teeth with your lips nearly shut, and slide along. Did you do it?)
Hooray! What a good try!

He said, 'When I am really good at this, I will hop from one fence to another, all along the way, from beginning to end.' Can you do that? 'Now,' he said, 'I will push this fence all along the way to see how strong I am.' And he did. He pushed those teeth, in front and behind, up and down. Clever Mr Tongue. Then he had another rest inside his mouth.

While he was inside, he heard a noise. What was it? He peeped around the left hand corner of the door. No one there. He peeped around the right hand corner of the door. No one there.

He looked down. Why there was Mr Chin! 'Hullo Mr Chin-Chin!'

He went in again and thought, 'I must do my exercises!'
(Pause)

Mr Tongue began to do his exercises. He stood in the middle of his house. He stretched up and pointed at the roof while somebody counted 1, 2, 3, and then he flopped down again.

He went outside, and pointed at Mr Nose, and then he flopped down again. He pointed at Mr Chin, while somebody counted 1, 2 ,3 and then he had another rest.

Now Mr Tongue stretched to touch the left hand corner of the lips, *(the gates)* and then the right hand corner, like this *(demonstrate)*. First he did it slowly, then he went faster. Then he had to have another rest. Soon it would be time for housework!

He had a list of things to do.
1. Polish the fences please, upstairs and downstairs.
2. Sweep the cobwebs off the ceiling, round and round.
3. Draw a straight line on the palate from the back door to the front door.
4. Now paint the gates, *(go round and round the top and bottom lips)*

Next, Mr Tongue had to do some sounds—this was speech work.
'PAH PAW POO, PAH PAY PEE, TAH TAW TOO, TAH TAY TEE, KAR KAW KOO, KAR KAY KEE.'

Sometimes he said them **fast,** and sometimes **slow,** or **loud** or **soft.** Then he had a big yawn and a stretch, towards the back door.

All the work was done. Now Mr Tongue could have a rest in his nice pink house.
(Pause)

When he finished resting, Mr Tongue wanted to draw. He wanted to draw a circle. He looked in the mirror.
(You draw a circle around your mouth with your finger.)

Next Mr Tongue tried to copy that circle: round and round the door
(your lips)
he went. Then he jumped up
(to the top lip)
and then down.
(bottom lip)

He saw a round hole in the ground
(make a round shape with your lips).
He heard a hissing noise. SSSSS.
(make the noise)
Who could it be? Out came a slippery snake!
(Show how it came out.)
Mr Tongue was so surprised that he hid in his house until somebody counted to 10. Then he came out, because he heard: ZZZZZ! He heard it again: ZZZZ! So he looked. Can you guess what it was? A bee buzzing. He was looking for a flower.
(Make a buzzing noise and find the way to a flower, any flower will do.)

Then Mr Tongue heard a strange sound: a clicking noise, a Skippy noise.

(Can you make it?)
Skippy Kangaroo was coming down the road.
(Click your tongue against the roof of your mouth. There are lots of different clicks you can make. Try!)

Here are more sounds to make, lots of times. These are lip sounds and they are very **short.**
PPPPP…a popping sound. (Do you like popcorn?)
BBBB…a loud banging, do it **loud,** then **soft.**

Now these are tongue sounds:
TTTTT…a sharp, soft tapping sound,
DDDD…a loud hammering sound. Mr Tongue heard a noise at the back door.
KKKKK…Who could it be? A kookaburra was tapping at the back door, can he come in?
GGGGG…Go away! This is Mr Tongue's house!
CH,CH,CH,…That was a train!
JJJ…JJJJ…JJJ…and that was a tractor. The kookaburra flew away.

Now, here are some **long** sounds made with the lips.
MMMMMMMMMMMMMMMMMMM
FFFFFFFFFFFFFFFFFFFFF, and
VVVVVVVVVVVV

Mr Tongue was really very tired now. He yawned,
AH, AH, AH,   AW, AW, AW   OH, OH, OH
OO, OO, OO   AH, AH, AH   AY, AY, AY
MMMMMMMMMMMMMMMMMMMMMM-
MMMMMM

Good Night!

EXERCISES FOR ADULTS

With older subjects, the tongue movements required in assessment of lingual proficiency can be taught more directly. The following exercises should be practiced every day for 5 to 10 minutes at a time both pre and post-operatively, until all lingual movements are proficient.

These simple exercises aim to increase tongue mobility and improve kinaesthetic sense in the oral cavity. They may be described to the patient as developing awareness of the connection between **planning** the movement, **feeling** the movement and **knowing** what the tongue, lips and palate are doing during a movement.

Visual and tactile feedback is as important with adults as it is with children, and the diagrams and the mirror should be used for as long as necessary.

Oral Kinaesthesia

1. Practising selected sounds, while sitting in front of a mirror, should include pointing to that part of the drawing which shows the active area of the oral musculature for each particular sound, and tapping it as the sound is said. Next, sounds should be practised in groups of two and three, gradually increasing the speed and continuing to coordinate the taps. This exercise will help in increasing diadochokinesis (DDK) rates but generalisation of these sounds into words should not be expected prematurely.

2. Viewing the oral musculature is an important ingredient of orientation in space. The patient is asked to open his mouth and look in the mirror, then close the mouth and touch a tooth, lip, cheek or the palate, as the speech pathologist points to it in the diagram. The patient then locates and touches one of his teeth with his tongue and identifies it as a front, back, upper or lower jaw or side tooth, by pointing to it on the diagram himself and verifying this with the mirror. Patients may then be asked to describe how they produce a chosen sound.

3. Make a chart of all the speech sounds. Ask the patient to time himself and repeat these sounds fast, slow, loud, soft, 10 times. He may then combine the sounds in chosen rhythms. (Familiar rhymes or songs make this exercise seem easier.)

4. The patient should practise producing the sounds in rhythm exercises. PP P PPP P PP varying the speed of the exercise. Next combine inflection and speed, in various combinations. Next, include varying the volume, and juggle fast/slow, loud/soft and high/low pitches, for different consonants.

5. Traditional DDK exercises may be extended to bring them within the scope of patients with tongue tie. When using the syllable 'PUH' only five repetitions at slow, then moderate then fast speeds should be requested. Next, reinforce the skill by using the same consonant with a variety of vowels, 'PUH,PUH,PUH, PEE,PEE,PEE, POO,POO, POO,' while pointing to the diagram of the vowel being elicited.

   When progressing to two consonants in two syllables, the sounds that are reminiscent of real words will be found to be more easily produced than nonsense syllables, for example 'PUHKUH' which sounds like 'pucker' will be easier to say than 'kuhpuh'. When attempting three consonants, e.g. 'PUHTUHKUH', pitch changes and a rolling rhythm will be found to facilitate this exercise.

6. The patient's name may be written in syllables, with a diagram of the oral musculature at each stage, and the name said, syllable by syllable, moving along the diagrams as the patient speaks.

7. This exercise may be repeated with any difficult word suggested by the patient.

8. A list may be made of 10 words, each starting with a plosive/nasal/sibilant/fricative or vowel, and practised using a mirror and concentrating on the characteristic qualities of the sound group. The patient should then listen to the speech pathologist say these sounds, exaggerating their distinctive qualities.

9. Tongue twisters may be used to reinforce rapid reiteration of sounds, but tongue twisters should not be performed at speed; instead the patient should start at a slow rate, and while visualising the alliterated letter, build up to speed gradually.

10. A taped word list of nonsense words, may be prepared where the vowel sounds AH, AY, EE, AI, ER, AW, OH, OO, are combined with any consonants. A diagram of the oral space and tongue posture for the relevant vowels should be referred to, as the patient goes slowly from one syllable to the other. Colour photographs of the mouth, showing lip postures for vowels have been most meaningful to patients with tongue tie, frequently being even more relevant that self monitoring with a mirror.

Tactile Input

1. The patient may put a piece of sticky food on the palate, then try to touch the spot where the food is with his tongue. This should be repeated several times. Improvement should be noted with practice. This exercise is described by Whitman and Rankow[26] and may easily be practised several times a day.

2. Correcting the infantile swallow should be done in stages and will take three to four lessons, although generalising the habit into spontaneous use will depend on altering the habit. As the patient swallows, the lower lip may be pulled aside to show the tongue in its incorrect thrusting position. Illustrate the correct position using tactile and visual input. Oral kinaesthesia depends on tactile feedback and memory. Visual feedback can serve to sensitise the patient to tactile feedback, hence the mirror is an indispensable aid to therapy with patients who have tongue tie.

3. To centralise tongue posture and reduce pressure on the top front teeth during infantile swallowing, the patient should practise EE, OO five times, with the tongue tip pressed against the bottom front teeth.

4. The patient should be drilled in stopping and starting the breath stream, while articulating continuant sounds, (i.e. F, V, S, Z, M, N, L, R, SH) without moving the articulators from their point of contact. Next, pairs of sounds should be practised so that the breathed and voiced qualities are contrasted, eg. F, V, S, Z, SH, ZH.

5. A short alliterated phrase, e.g. 'Bobby's big blue balloon burst' may be used. Before saying the phrase, the speech pathologist shows the patient a drawing of the posture for the bilabial sound. Using the drawing, modelling the lip contact with hand gesture, and giving a verbal description, the patient is

asked to say the phrase, while impressing the image of bilabial closure on his mind.

6. Using a mirror for visual feedback, the patient should protrude and point the tongue, then broaden and narrow it alternately. When this has been mastered, the patient should try to change the shape of the oral aperture by spreading or pointing the lips, and maintaining the pointed or broad shape of the tongue.

7. After looking at a drawing of the oral space, the patient should attempt the following movements with his tongue: trace the outline of the teeth, upper and lower, front and back, explore the hard palate, and reach back towards the soft palate.

8. While the pictorial representation may be used to facilitate the exercise initially, eventually the patient should be asked to do the exercise with his eyes closed.

Rhythm

1. Work on syllables. Make 10-word charts of one, two, three, and four-syllable words, and show the patient how to use stress in polysyllabic words to make them easier to pronounce. Show him how to make syllables more forceful by squeezing the stomach muscles, rather than forcing from the larynx. Use tapping or colour coding to distinguish the stressed and unstressed syllables, which these patients will otherwise have great difficulty in discerning.

2. Devise an auditory discrimination task that requires the patient to listen to polysyllabic words and identify the strongest syllable, by tapping out the rhythm. Next, repeat the exercise without tapping out the rhythm.

3. A metronome, or the rhythm of a familiar song with a strong beat may be used to reinforce tongue exercises. For instance have the patient move the tongue strongly from the left to the right hand corner of the mouth precisely, in time to Baa Baa Black Sheep, or some other two-beat rhyme.

Speed and Intonation

1. Introduce speed, volume and pitch changes, in two or three-word phrases, and extend these to longer utterances, while still varying loudness, rapidity and inflection. Use tapping and rhythm to assist the patient in speeding up responses.

2. Use exercises involving rapid verbal responses to speech and have the patient respond speedily. Later, use variations of speed in reading or speaking, to show how meaning can be changed thereby. Teach the use of pauses to change meaning and increase impact of the spoken words.

3. Practise varying intonation for 'happy, sad, angry, frightened, tired,' sentences. Ask the patient to make up his own sentence to match an emotion. Show him how his own utterances can be made more effective, by using flexible changes of tone.

4. Read an expressive passage with exaggerated variations of intonation. Identify pitch changes and discuss their implication. Read the passage again with different intonation and discuss what the changes imply. Next ask the patient to read the passage as he chooses.

Continuous Speech Exercises

1. Read a passage, and tape record it as a model for the patient. Colour code the sentences as

loud, soft, fast, slow. Play the tape again. Have the patient follow the code, and read the same passage with the tape recording. Discuss.

2. Combine these aspects of speech in exercises, using a short sentence, and variations of stress, volume, pitch and speed. Read a short sentence aloud, changing either stress, loudness, pitch or speed, in one word, and ask the patient to identify the word that was different, describe or identify the difference, then attempt to reproduce it.

3. Add intonation onto other practice sentences to demonstrate the resulting differences in meaning. Practising only three or four sample sentences will be found to be quite effective in showing the patient how to use pitch, volume, and speed changes to good effect in connected speech.

4. Monitor the patient's ability to maintain error free utterance in reading, reciting or speaking continuously for a maximum period of 5 minutes.

5. Make a 'hard word' list. Teach these words using colour coding for stress and syllabification, and gradually say the words faster; next, include them in a sentence.

References

1. Greene JS. Anomalies of the speech mechanism and associated voice and speech disorders. N York J Med 1945; 45(6): 605–608.

2. Oldfield MC. Tongue-tie. BMJ 1959; 2: 1181–1182.

3. Ketty N, Sciullo PA. Ankyloglossia with psychological implications. ASDC J Dent Child 1974; 4: 43–46.

4. DePorte JV, Parkhurst E. Congenital malformation and birth injuries among the children born in New York state outside of New York city from 1940–1942. N York J Med 1945; 45(9): 1097–1100.

5. McEnery ET, Gaines FP. Tongue-tie in infants and children. J Pediatr 1941; 18: 252–255.

6. Schaumann BF, Peagler FD, Gorlin RJ. Minor craniofacial anomalies among a Negro population: II Prevalence of tongue anomalies. Oral Surgery 1970; 29(5): 729–734.

7. Witkop CJ. Genetics and dentistry. Eugen Q 1958; 5(1): 15–22.

8. Williams WN, Waldron CM. Assessment of lingual function when ankyloglossia (tongue-tie) is suspected. J Am Dent Assoc 1985; 110: 353–356.

9. Wright JE. Tongue-tie. J Paediatr Child Health 1995; 31(4): 276–278.

10. Fletcher SG, Meldrum JR. Lingual function and relative length of the lingual frenulum. J Speech Hear Res 1968; 11(2): 382–390.

11. Pechey J. A general treatise of the diseases of infants and children. 1697: 91–93. Extract reproduced in J Hum Lact 1990; 6(3): 134.

12. Cullum IM. Nova et vetera: An old wives' tale. BMJ 1959; 2: 497–498.

13. Kingston MH. The woman warrior—memoirs of a girlhood among ghosts. London: Picador, 1981: 148.

14. van der Waal I. Diseases of the tongue. Chicago: Quintessence Publishing Company Inc, 1986: 21.

15. Browne D. Tongue-tie. BMJ 1959; 2: 952.

16. Mortensen K, Connelly M. Breastfeeding through the ages: Part III Advice to mothers in the twentieth century. NMAA Newsletter Sept/Oct 1994: 18–19.

17. Block JR. The role of the speech clinician in determining indications for frenulotomy in cases of ankyloglossia. N Y State Dent J 1968; 34: 479–481.

18. Morley ME. The development and disorders of speech in childhood. London: Churchill Livingstone, 1972: 420–421.

19. Wallace AF. Tongue tie. Lancet 1963; 2: 377–378.

20. Kern I. Tongue tie. Med J Aust 1991; 155: 33–34.

21. Barclay JK. Release of tongue-tie. Australia Patient Management 1990; 14(8): 21–24.

22. McDonald M. Private correspondence. 1991.

23. Thorley Phillips V. Correcting faulty suck: tongue protrusion and the breastfed infant. Med J Aust 1992; 156: 508.

24. Notestine GE. The importance of the identification of ankyloglossia (short lingual frenulum) as a cause of breastfeeding problems. J Hum Lact 1990; 6(3): 113–115.

25. Ketty N. Ankyloglossia with periodontal manifestations. (unpub.)
26. Whitman CL, Rankow RM. Diagnosis and management of ankyloglossia. Am J Orthod Dentofacial Orthop 1961; 47(6): 423–438.
27. Dworkin JP, Culatta RA. Tongue strength: its relationship to tongue thrusting, open-bite, and articulatory proficiency. J Speech & Hear Dis 1980; 45: 277–282.
28. Young EC, Sacks GK. Examining for tongue tie. Clin Pediatr (Phila) 1979; 18 (5): 298.
29. Jones PG. Clinical paediatric surgery: diagnosis and management. 2nd ed. Oxford, Blackwell Scientific Publications, 1976: 188.
30. Douglas BL, Kresberg H. Surgical correction of ankyloglossia. N Y State Dent J 1954; 20(10): 477–479.
31. Tuerk M, Lubit EC. Ankyloglossia. Plast Reconstr Surg 1959; 24: 271–276.
32. Rogers JG, Douglas BL. Surgical correction of ankyloglossia. U S Armed Forces Med J 1952; 3(5): 695–697.

Glossary

Aetiological—causal.

Agenesis—incomplete and imperfect development.

Alveolus—tooth socket.

Ankyloglossia (tongue tie)—a condition where the fold of tissue connecting the undersurface of the tongue with the floor of the mouth (the frenum linguae) is too short.

Aspiration—inhalation of fluid or food particles into the lungs.

Bilabial—pertaining to both lips.

Buccal—pertaining to cheek or mouth.

DDK—see diadochokinesis.

Deglutition—the act or process of swallowing.

Diadochokinesis—the normal ability to make voluntary reiterated movements at varying rates of speed.

Dorsum—the back of an organ.

Dysphonia—disorder of phonation, an abnormality of the sound of the voice.

Dyspraxia—disorder in the performance of voluntary movement, in the absence of paralysis.

Encopretic—faecal incontinence at an age when sphincter control may be expected.

Endotracheal—within the trachea or windpipe.

Eneuresis—urinary incontinence at an age when sphincter control may be expected.

Edentulous—without teeth.

Epithelioma—a growth arising in epithelial tissue, usually skin.

Fibrosed—hardened by the formation of excessive fibrous tissue.

Frenectomy—removal of a portion of the frenum.

Frenulotomy—incision of the frenulum.

Frenulum—see frenum.

Fraenum—see frenum.

Frenum (frenum linguae)—a fold of membrane which limits the movement of an organ. It stretches from the undersurface of the tongue in the midline, to the floor of the mouth. Also fraenum, frenulum, phraenum and phrenum.

Genioglossus (glossa)—the musculature of the tongue.

Haemophilia—an inherited bleeding disorder, which causes prolonged bleeding, after even minor injuries.

Hyperplasia—increase in size or bulk of a body, as a result of increase in cell number.

Hypersalivation—excessive secretion of saliva.

Incontinent—lacking control.

Kinaesthesia—sensory impulses underlying muscle tension and posture which control and correlate the position, in relation to each other, of muscles, joints and muscle groups.

Lateralisation—away from the median line, at, or to, the side.

Larynx—the voice box, situated at the upper end of the trachea, below and in front of the pharynx.

Lingual—pertaining to the tongue.

Lisping—the dentalising of sibilant sounds, so that they are incorrectly produced by contact with the upper front teeth.

Macroglossia—an abnormally large tongue.

Malocclusion—faulty alignment (of the teeth and jaws).

Mandibular—pertaining to the lower jaw.

Mastication—the act of chewing.

Maxillary—pertaining to the upper jaw.

Morphology—the form or structure of a living thing.

Myofunctional—pertaining to the functioning of a muscle.

Nasality—pertaining to the quality of speech. May refer to either insufficient, excessive or mixed nasal resonance.

Nasopharynx—that part of the pharynx which is above the soft palate, and inside the nasal cavity.

Oromuscular—pertaining to the muscles of the mouth.

Pharynx—the cavity at the back of the mouth, consisting of oropharynx and nasopharynx.

Phrenum—see frenum

Sibilants—sounds characterised by a hissing or whistling quality. In speech, this applies to S, Z, SH and 'SURE' as in 'pleasure'.

Sulci—furrows or grooves.

Tongue-thrust—the constant protrusion of the tongue beyond the gums and teeth.

Uvula—the central tag-like structure hanging down from the soft palate.

Vermilion—the junction of the skin and the red part of the lips.

Z-Plasty—a surgical procedure, where the incision made is in the shape of a 'Z', providing scope for stretching.

Index

A
alveolar ridge 38-40, 75

B
behaviour 11, 14-16, 23, 26, 35, 44, 55, 58, 59, 63

C
cerebral palsy 10,19, 26, 29, 38, 39, 56, 57, 63
cleft
   lip 26, 29, 32
   palate 1, 10, 28, 29, 48, 49, 63
cosmetic appearance 7, 11, 32, 53, 62, 64

D
deglutition 12
delayed intervention 6
dental hygiene 9, 13, 22, 65
developmental delay 17, 29, 39, 40, 63
diadochokinesis (DDK) 32, 35, 67, 79
diadochokinetic 3, 18, 35
diathermy 31, 72, 73
dribble 33, 44, 65
dyspraxia 20, 35

E
emotional disturbances 26, 39
epithelioma 12

F
feeding
   assessment of 65
   bottle 5, 20
   breast 5, 7, 8, 14, 20, 22, 27, 28, 30, 37, 58, 65
   habits 35, 65
   skills 57, 62, 65

G
grooved director 4

H
haemophilia 29
hearing loss 29, 39, 40
hyperplasia 29
hypersalivation 7, 22, 33, 65

I
infantilising 37
infants 4, 8, 22, 28, 30, 31

L
lactation consultant 8
lingual
   grooving 23
   limitation of movement 23, 60
   movement 2, 9, 10, 15, 18, 22, 23, 36, 44, 50, 51, 53, 58, 62, 79

M
malnourishment 5
malocclusion 10, 25, 38, 48
mandibular prognathism 38
mastication 12, 37, 10
mastitis 8, 58, 65
mucobuccal fold 42, 50, 54, 60, 66

N
nipples 8, 22, 65

O
oral
  hygiene 9, 19, 22, 25, 27, 37, 48, 49, 51, 52,
    61-63, 65
  kinaesthesia 9, 14, 27, 33, 34, 36, 37, 39, 40, 47,
    48, 50, 51, 58, 60, 62, 65, 68, 69, 75

R
regurgitation 9

S
self esteem 14, 26, 61
speech
  defects 2, 20, 26, 63
  dysphonia 13
  fluency 12, 13, 40, 68
  impairment 7
  pronunciation 7, 12, 40, 51, 57, 59, 60
  quality of 7, 19, 68
sublingual cysts 1
supra bulbar palsy 35
surgery
  recovery after 32, 33, 39, 42, 61
  snipping 30
  sutures 30, 32, 36, 72, 73

T
tactile 39, 75, 80
TAP 17, 19, 20, 27, 41, 62-64, 69, 70
tongue
  dimpling of 22, 64
  medial lingual grooving 23
  mobility 79
  movements
    circumlocution 24, 25, 42, 48, 50
    lateral 9, 24, 42, 52, 66
    pointing 22-24, 37, 38, 40, 44, 54, 66
  notching 21, 23, 24, 38, 64
  positions
    elevation 10, 17, 24, 38, 39, 42, 57, 64, 66
    protrusion 2, 6, 10, 12, 19, 22, 23, 24, 42, 48,
      54, 58, 60, 66
    retraction 10, 16, 56, 60, 67
tongue tie
  definition 1, 2
  incidence of 1, 2, 5
  prevalence 1, 3, 5
  surgery for 5, 28, 31, 32, 57
  untreated 2, 4, 50
tongue-tip
  agenesis of the 18, 22, 35
  hypoplasia of the 35

V
vermilion 2, 24, 54, 56, 58, 66
visual assessment 20
voice quality 26